Picture Yourself Dancing:

Step-by-Step Instruction for Ballroom, Latin, Country, and More

Shawn and Joanna Trautman

THOMSON

COURSE TECHNOLOGY

Professional ■ Technical ■ Reference

ISBN: 1-59863-246-9

Library of Congress Catalog Card Number: 2006923269

Printed in the United States of America

06 07 08 09 10 BU 10 9 8 7 6 5 4 3 2 1

Thomson Course Technology PTR,
a division of Thomson Learning Inc.
25 Thomson Place
Boston, MA 02210
http://www.courseptr.com

THOMSON

COURSE TECHNOLOGY

Professional ■ Technical ■ Reference

Publisher and General Manager, Thomson Course Technology PTR:
Stacy L. Hiquet

Associate Director of Marketing:
Sarah O'Donnell

Manager of Editorial Services:
Heather Talbot

Marketing Manager:
Heather Hurley

Acquisitions Editor:
Megan Belanger

Project Editor/Copy Editor:
Cathleen D. Snyder

PTR Editorial Services Coordinator:
Elizabeth Furbish

Interior Layout:
Shawn Morningstar

Cover Designer:
Mike Tanamachi

Indexer:
Katherine Stimson

To our daughters, McKenzie and Breanna.
We already love to dance with you and are
inspired in our instruction by the two of you.

Acknowledgments

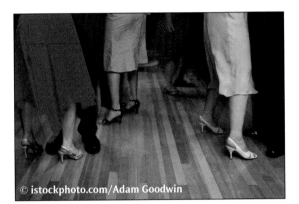

© istockphoto.com/Adam Goodwin

THIS BOOK WAS truly a team effort. We would like to especially thank Ginger Trautman for her research, creativity, and critical input—we couldn't have done it without you! Many thanks to Nancy Dollar as well as Bruce and Ginger Trautman for the many hours of running after our toddler and helping us care for our newborn as we wrote this book. A special thanks to Shannon McKnight for her continued support and wonderful picture-taking abilities. You're the best!.Thanks also to Dan Salafia for all his tireless efforts in helping our DVD come to life. Keep up the great work! Thank you to Megan Belanger for approaching us with this wonderful opportunity, as well as cheering us on through the writing process. Thanks to Cathleen Snyder and Shawn Morningstar, who took our text and created the beautiful book that you are reading now. Finally, thank you to all of our friends, family, students, and fellow dancers who allowed us to include their pictures in this book and for their continued support.

About the Authors

SHAWN TRAUTMAN is a consultant, corporate trainer, choreographer, and public speaker on many different forms of lead-and-follow dance, as well as line dancing. He is the director of operations for Xpress Innovations, Inc., where his days are filled with editing and producing instructional DVDs, teaching both private and group classes, and designing curricula.

In addition to holding an MBA in organizational leadership and communication, where he focused on training the trainers. Shawn has been a coach and mentor to numerous world champions as well as countless social dancers since 1991. Shawn welcomes people from all walks of life to his classes, regardless of shape, size, or ability. His broad experience in both dance and advanced learning techniques makes his methods of instruction innovative, easy, and fun.

JOANNA TRAUTMAN is currently a stay-at-home mother of two and a graduate student pursuing her MBA in technological management. Although caring for her daughters now consumes the bulk of her days, Joanna continues to assist with business analysis and marketing for Xpress Innovations, Inc. She also teaches both private and group classes and is instrumental in the filming and content of the company's DVDs.

SHAWN AND JOANNA TRAUTMAN teach live classes in and around the Tampa Bay area in Florida, where they've helped tens of thousands of students attain goals. Whether it's giving someone the confidence to step foot on a dance floor for the very first time, go to their first line dance class in a country-western nightclub, dance at their dream wedding reception, or even compete at championship levels, Shawn and Joanna have proven they have what it takes to quickly and efficiently bring success to their students. Through a strong emphasis on the basic mechanical components of each dance in combination with clear communication between the dance partners, their instruction has made the difference for their students.

In addition to live instruction, Shawn and Joanna have created and produced a complete line of instructional DVDs. In an effort to take their instruction beyond the studio and into the living rooms of their students, the DVD collection continues to reach more and more students who would not otherwise learn to dance due to various reasons, such as geographic difficulties for live classes or simple discomfort about going to a studio for a private or group lesson. To contact Shawn and Joanna directly, whether for their DVDs or for teaching, coaching, consulting, or other reasons, call 1-877-DANCE-01 (1-877-32623-01) or visit the Web site www.ShawnTrautman.com.

Table of Contents

Chapter 5   Picture Yourself Two-Stepping 105

Chapter 6   Picture Yourself Swing Dancing 125

Chapter 10   Picture Yourself Dancing the West Coast Swing 219

Introduction

LEARNING TO DANCE through a book has always proven challenging at best...until now. Welcome to *Picture Yourself Dancing*, a comprehensive book and DVD combination that gets straight to the heart of what beginners need.

When we began to write *Picture Yourself Dancing*, we were faced with the daunting task of taking our curriculum from our beginner classes and putting it in book form to accompany an instructional DVD. Our goal in writing this book was to give novice dancers a tool that, if used as directed, would teach them the basics of each dance so they could get out on the social dance floor and have some fun. We also wanted to set dancers up for success should they continue to pursue any of the dances with further classes, lessons, or instructional videos or DVDs.

Picture Yourself Dancing isn't one of those books that shows pictures of supermodel-like dancers posing with no true instruction, because we believe dancing is for everyone, and most people who enjoy social dancing have average figures and are not in Olympian shape. This book is not one of those guides that has countless terms and definitions that you'll never use, nor does it expect you to learn to dance from an artist's rendition of steps on a floor with imaginary lines that, to the untrained eye, look like the remnants of a ball of yarn after an attack by a playful kitten. The approach we took to writing this book was to separate the essential building blocks from all the clutter and introduce them in an order that makes sense for beginners.

In addition to the clear, concise instructions in the book, we've chosen to include and integrate one of our bestselling DVDs with this book. The DVD, a 75-minute visual reference, covers everything from the four connection points, to tips for leaders and followers, to the basics of eight different dances that are included in this book. We wrote *Picture Yourself Dancing* to be synchronized with the curriculum taught in the DVD. As you continue to explore this text, you will find that we refer to the DVD frequently.

As you read this introduction, you are preparing yourself to embark on an exciting journey of learning to dance. *Picture Yourself Dancing* is truly one of a kind because it focuses on thinking patterns and true lead-and-follow dancing. Whether mastery of social dancing has been a lifelong dream or you are simply trying to learn a few moves to impress or meet someone special, this book is for you.

To really start out on the right foot, it is important that you master the foundational concepts taught in Chapter 2, "Beginner Basics." From there, you can either pick and choose the dances that you want to learn, or you can work your way straight through the text. The basics of couples dancing can easily be learned; however, you must have a proper foundation from which to work.

We look forward to seeing you out on the dance floor after you've had a chance to do some quick learning with our book and DVD. Don't spend all of your time trying to perfect it at home—get out and dance with others, take additional classes, experiment with moves, and find ways to have fun and enjoy your new hobby. A lifetime of enjoyment awaits you!

—Shawn and Joanna Trautman

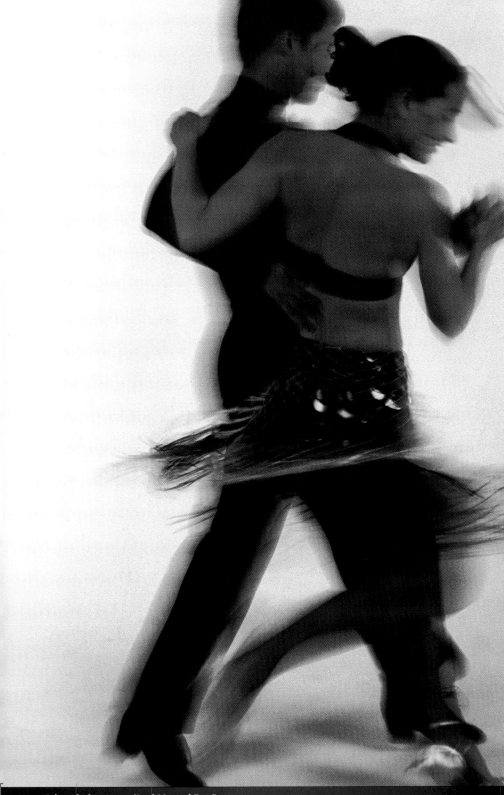

Dance Floor *Impressions*

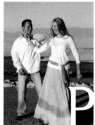

PICTURE YOURSELF floating across the floor to an elegant waltz or spinning past your partner like a whirling dervish to the driving beat of a West coast swing. Visualize yourself maneuvering your partner around the dance floor to an upbeat two-step or sweeping your partner off her feet, figuratively, during a romantic slow dance. Hold onto these images of success in couples dancing as you dive into your introduction to couples social dancing.

If the first two sentences of this paragraph left you saying to yourself, "Wow, that sounds great, but what does a waltz look like?" or something similar, hang on—this chapter was written for you. For those readers who already have a smattering of dance experience (enough that you feel confident in your learning goals), do read on because this first chapter will provide invaluable groundwork for your dance education. In this chapter, we will explore the synergy of advanced learning techniques and dance floor basics that will jumpstart your dancing, and we will examine the world and etiquette of social couples dancing.

Introduction to Social Dancing

SOCIAL DANCING encompasses a wide variety of couples dances, as well as various styles of dancing. In general terms, social dancing includes everything from the hot and spicy salsa to the top-notch two-step and all the classics in between, such as the foxtrot, swing, and waltz. Basically, social couples dances include all dances that are performed with a partner, in contrast to dances such as line dancing, which does not require a partner.

Another unique attribute of the social dance family is along the same vein as the first, but takes it a step further. Social dances are not just performed with a partner; the successful execution of the dance depends on the interpersonal communication between the partners during the dance, which is commonly referred to as the *lead-and-follow* aspect of the dance.

Other dance forms, such as ballet, modern, and jazz, can be performed as partner dances, but they are also perfectly acceptable and equally beautiful when performed solo. The artist's intrapersonal communication and interpretation of the music are the defining attributes of these dances.

In contrast, a solo foxtrot is merely a dancer progressing around a dance floor in a box-step pattern without a partner to initiate or complete the led patterns associated with the dance, leaving a relatively meaningless series of rhythmic steps taking the solo dancer around a circle. Hence the term *social dancing* because it is based on a temporary social relationship formed between two partners strictly for the purpose of completing the dance at hand.

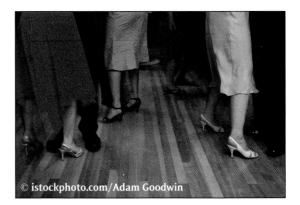
© istockphoto.com/Adam Goodwin

If you do not currently have a dance partner, do not be dismayed; a high percentage of beginning social dancers start out in the same situation. The beauty of lead-and-follow social dancing is that the basics of each dance can be learned individually for application in a mixed social setting. Once you are properly armed with the basics of a particular dance, you should be ready to dance with a corresponding leader or follower who also knows the standardized basic steps of the same dance.

Many people learn to dance for the sole purpose of meeting people of the opposite sex. History has proven this to be a successful and palatable strategy because those individuals who can dance have a perceived "edge" on the competition due to their newly acquired musical sense and comfort on the dance floor, as well as a real advantage created by the confidence instilled by simply knowing how to dance and subsequently behave in a potentially awkward social occasion.

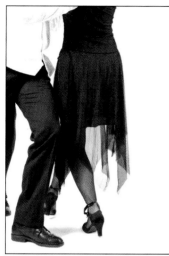

© istockphoto.com/Paul Piebinga

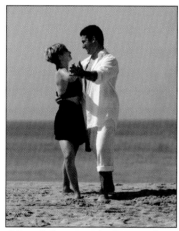

© istockphoto.com/Galina Barskaya

As you learn the basics of the various dances, picture yourself practicing your newly acquired dance skills to different styles of music at venues across the globe. Keep in mind that the footwork and the lead-and-follow aspect of each dance are consistent in every situation in every corner of the world, despite music, surroundings, and attire.

Though there are rules of etiquette associated with social dancing, please do not be intimidated or fall victim to the misconception that social dancing is exclusive, elitist, unattainable, or stuffy. Once you understand these rules, which will be broken down later in this chapter and fleshed out through the rest of the book, you will leave the most pretentious in the dust as you step confidently onto the dance floor in any situation.

By the same token, as you pursue a social dance education, your journey may take you to several places and groups of people. Social dancing is practiced worldwide and can be learned through private lessons, group lessons, or self-instruction methods, such as this book and DVD combination, or simply by imitation if the individual is so inclined. Each method has its own unique advantages, and individual preferences and learning styles play critical roles. Whether your dance education takes you to the level of a competent social dancer or your desire to compete launches you into the realm of competition, performance, and DanceSport, a firm foundation in the essentials is critical. However, your dancing goals will determine your dance education.

As we will discuss later in this chapter and reinforce throughout the book, social dancing is a very large umbrella covering a wide variety of dances, music styles, and situations. Although appropriate at a black-tie event where the menu includes champagne and caviar, the waltz is also appropriate in a country-western nightclub where beer on tap is the beverage of choice.

The various types of dance education and their benefits and drawbacks will be discussed at further length later in this chapter, as well as criteria to look for when selecting the instruction method appropriate to your goals and budget, whether it be a self-instruction method, such as the book you are currently reading, or a highly specialized dance coach for learning acrobatic lifts and stunts for international competition.

Rapid Learning Using the Book/DVD Combo (Visual, Audio, and Kinesthetic)

IF YOU'RE READY for a new, innovative, and exciting dance-training program that represents a dramatic departure from traditional dance instruction as it is currently known, then this book and DVD combo is perfect for you. Auditory (audio), visual, and kinesthetic (physical) learning styles are all combined in this package to give you the best possible dance instruction that will have you dancing in just a couple of short hours...and we're not talking about looking like you can dance, we're talking about real lead-and-follow dancing. Unique features of this dance-training program include:

▶ **A thorough step-by-step four-color visual introduction to nine different social dances**

▶ **Sections in each chapter that separate out leader's and follower's footwork**

▶ **A six-W approach to each dance that quickly delivers the who, what, where, when, why, and wear of each dance**

▶ **Full integration, including references, with a best-selling 75-minute beginner instructional DVD from the Shawn Trautman *Learn to Dance* series**

This unique dance-training program narrows the scope down to what's essential for learning, starting with the incorporation of the three learning styles.

Speaking of the different learning styles, most people remember only about 20 percent of what they read, yet they remember closer to 60 percent of what they physically do. It's been said, however, that the average person remembers 90 percent of what they see, hear, say, and do. If you just read

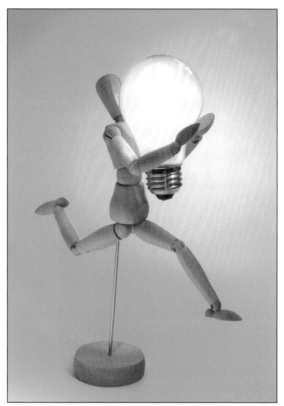

© istockphoto.com/Elena Ray

this book, chances are you would be cheating yourself out of most of its value. For this reason, the visual *Picture Yourself* series has taken this approach to learning. By introducing what learners need in an order that makes logical sense and by utilizing multi-sensory teaching techniques, this unique book and DVD combination enables learners who pace themselves and use the combo as instructed to achieve rapid results that won't quickly be forgotten. Each of the senses carries its own unique attributes for learning, and most people are inclined to use one more than the others.

Regardless, the easier information is to process and assimilate, the better it will stay in your long-term memory. Next, we'll look at each of the senses individually, as well as how they're portrayed in this dance-training program.

Visual

This book is a visual experience by definition; however, there are a few signature components of this learning experience that can create an environment for success for a visual learner. Take note in the following sections of the tools included to enhance your visual learning experience.

Written Word

This book incorporates a unique "six-W" approach to each dance that covers the who, what, where, when, why, and wear to quickly get you situated on the right foot. Look for the six Ws at the beginning of each dance, and you'll find out *who* dances the dance, *what* the dance is, *where* the dance is typically done, *when* is the right time to dance the dance, *why* the dance is danced, and what to *wear* when you go out to dance it.

Pictures

The pictures in *Picture Yourself Dancing* were specifically selected and staged to provide clear snapshot demonstrations of points emphasized in the text and highlighted in the DVD. Sometimes a still shot allows learners to hone in on one particular aspect of a lead or foot position that was otherwise escaping them. Sometimes that one individual detail makes the difference between complete success and frustration for a student. Another advantage of the pictures being integrated with the text is that for many visual learners, the learning process is more like a storyboard of sequential pictures when this teaching method is used.

Step-by-Step Descriptions

For all of our learners out there who must have special requests or to-do lists written down for a visual record, or for whom the request or task is long forgotten minutes after it is mentioned, we have included step-by-step descriptions for each of the moves, positions, concepts, and so on throughout the book. This is for your reference reinforcement following DVD instruction and practice, as well as your initial learning process.

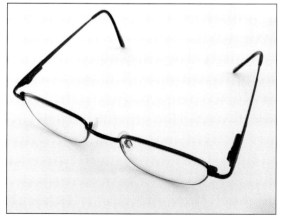

© istockphoto.com/Duncan Walker

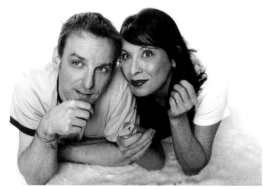

© istockphoto.com/Lise Gagne

DVD: Watch Body Movements

Last but certainly not least, the *Picture Yourself Dancing* learning program includes a 75-minute instructional DVD. For all of you visual learners out there, make good use of your pause, rewind, and slow-motion features on your DVD player. The DVD is filmed with picture-in-picture from multiple camera angles to provide as complete a picture of the instructors and moves as possible.

Auditory

Although this is a book, you can enhance your auditory learning experience by employing the learning practices in the following sections.

Memorize the Steps Aloud

For you auditory learners who are learning to dance from a book, stimulate your auditory learning processes by memorizing dance steps aloud. Repeating key steps or rhythms aloud while reading and then practicing will greatly expedite the learning process and cement key principles in your long-term muscle memory. By involving just one more of the five senses in the learning process, you will dramatically increase your information retention.

This advanced learning technique is probably as old as the hills, but it falls into the category of "tried and true." Implementation of this technique is as simple as saying aloud to yourself and your partner rhythm patterns, such as "quick, quick, slow, slow" as you learn and practice the two-step, or "step, touch, step, touch, step, touch" as you practice your smooth slow dance. As you progress into more advanced dances and move sequences, you will find this technique very helpful as you seek ways to keep your place in the dance's basic pattern.

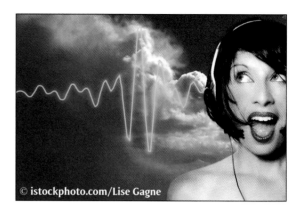

© istockphoto.com/Lise Gagne

Hear Instruction on the DVD

One of the major advantages of the combination of written and digital media in the *Picture Yourself Dancing* learning experience is the audiovisual aspect of the enclosed DVD. As you progress through the written instructions in this book, you will hear the instructors, Shawn and Joanna Trautman, breaking down the same moves on the DVD. For the auditory learning experience, this is a huge combination jump-start and reinforcement tool for the learning process. It will behoove some learners to watch the segment first on the DVD, then read and work through the written text, and then practice with the DVD. For others, the DVD will serve as a reinforcement tool only, following a visual and verbal analysis of the written textual instruction. You are the best person to determine the most powerful learning sequence as you work through *Picture Yourself Dancing*.

Dance to the Music on the DVD

Lest we forget one of the key components to a successful dance, this is a good place to remind ourselves about the music to which we are dancing. As you watch and practice with the DVD, listen to the music. The music used on the DVD has been carefully selected based on beat pattern, speed, style, and "danceability." None of the songs on the DVD have lyrics, which reduces the distraction created when one or both of the dance partners cannot resist the urge to sing along with the song. Remember, you should be using your voice to practice beat patterns, steps, and other key concepts aloud. As you practice with the DVD, try to allow the speed and style of the music to saturate your memory

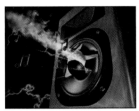

so you can recall the type of music that goes with a particular dance when you are out dancing at a ballroom, wedding, or nightclub.

© istockphoto.com/Slavoljub Pantelic

Kinesthetic

Learning to dance is a physical activity, but the kinesthetic aspects of this learning experience start before you get on the dance floor and expand beyond the studio.

Write It Down

Kinesthetic learning is at the heart of dance instruction. This isn't a huge surprise because kinesthetic learning provides the umbrella for all "hands-on," activity-based educational experiences. What might surprise you as a learner is where and when the kinesthetic learning starts. Activate the kinesthetic portion of your brain and memory by engaging in the multi-sensory experience of taking notes as you read this book and watch the DVD. Not only will you be providing yourself with an additional written record or cue card to stimulate your visual learning, you will also be engaging the activity-hungry portion of your brain with the act of note-taking.

Exercises

Several places beginning in Chapter 2 will highlight exercises to assist you in developing particular muscular traits or dance habits. Note these exercises and incorporate them into your routine at home.

For example, in Chapter 2, an abbreviated series of stretching exercises is outlined. These gentle exercises, if you are physically capable of performing them, are beneficial as you pursue your daily activities as well as learn to dance.

Drills

Throughout the instructional chapters on each of the individual dances, as well as the introductory section on dance floor basics, you will see drills noted. Very simply put, *practice the drills*. The *Picture Yourself Dancing* book and the accompanying DVD are specifically designed to be cumulative learning experiences. Success in the major cumulative concepts taught in this book and DVD is achieved through mastering the individual components of couples social dancing and the individual dances.

Dancing along with the DVD

As stressed in the visual and auditory learning sections, use the DVD. Dance along with the instructors as they go through the curriculum. You can watch the DVD first to take notes and absorb, but it is imperative that at some point in your learning experience you get up, get moving, and start dancing along with the DVD. This will stimulate the activity-based portions of your brain, much like note-taking, but on a more systemic level, and it will give you a chance to practice making your body do what the instructor's body is doing as he or she is doing it.

Practice and Muscle Memory

Finally, practice, practice, practice. Practice, with and without the DVD, will begin to establish the necessary muscle memory to transfer the dancing basics learned from your short-term memory to your long-term memory. Practice in the comfort of your own home, practice tapping rhythms to various radio stations as you drive around, and practice your alignment and carriage as you stand, sit, and ambulate about your daily activities.

Always check with your healthcare provider before starting this or any other fitness or physical activity program.

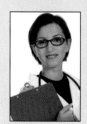 **Each individual's ability to perform all activities presented in this or any other fitness program is best determined by that individual and his or her healthcare provider.**

© istockphoto.com/Dmitry Obukhov

Putting It All Together

Effective learning starts with a confident and motivated mindset toward the material at hand. If you're not relaxed and open to the material, the best teaching techniques in the world won't help you. Next, you'll want to absorb the dance training in the way that best suits your learning preference, whether it's visual, auditory, kinesthetic, or a combination of the three. After absorbing the material, you'll want to explore the material to the extent that you turn your newly learned skills into a deep understanding. You can do this by digging deeper into each subject area and by asking questions of those around you. Look up information online or go to local classes or dances and ask questions. The more your mind is involved, the easier it'll be for your body to pick the dances up. Memorizing key sequences, numbers, facts, or steps is another way to quickly turn this dance-training program into a long-term foundation. Most of all, you'll want to demonstrate that you know the material. Get out and dance. Practice, practice, practice, as they say, but do so only with the right information because muscle memory is hard to break. Dance with others and continue your learning. You're embarking upon a whole new world of opportunities, and you don't want to go into it the wrong way.

To make the most of your learning experience, you'll want to go through and read this chapter and the next at length to make sure you understand them. Combine your reading with the first lesson on the DVD and get your first taste of the visual, audio, and kinesthetic styles working together. From that point forward, it's best to just dive into each dance and spend time understanding it, watching it on the DVD, and then dancing it yourself. Celebrate your successes along the way, and you'll keep the momentum up until you get through the final dance. If you've never danced before, it'll definitely behoove you to start with the slow dance section after you've completed Chapters 1 and 2 and are comfortable with the dance floor basics. The basics that you'll learn in Chapter 2 are essential for all dances and will forever be in your arsenal as you move into the dance scene. If you bypass the fundamentals taught in Chapter 2 of this book and go directly into the dances, you'll dramatically increase the amount of time it'll take you to go from being someone who has never danced to being a socially adept dancer who's the life of the party.

Formal versus Informal

A S WE HAVE ALREADY discussed, social dancing can be and is practiced in a broad spectrum of settings, ranging from the extremely formal ball or rigid competition to the impromptu slow dance on a beach during an inspiring sunset. Social dancing has made a place in myriad activities in contemporary Western culture.

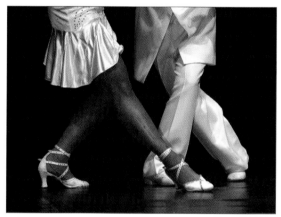

© istockphoto.com/Daniel Ruta

Formal

The images that usually come to mind first when the term "ballroom dancing" is mentioned are couples swirling around the floor in bright and bejeweled costumes with rigid posture and regal carriage. This highly formal and stylized version of social dancing is usually reserved for ballroom competitions, performances, and the movies. This is the haute couture of the social dancing world.

The majority of the dancing that you see and practice in this realm is choreographed, as opposed to spontaneous lead-and-follow dancing, which will be discussed later in this chapter. This is the world in which the proverbial big bucks are spent in instruction, costuming, performance, and all-around lifestyle.

For some dancers, this enclave of the dancing world is a nirvana; however, for the majority of the dancing community and beginner dancers, this most formal end of the spectrum of social dancing is rather remote.

For some potential dancers, the image of the stylized formal ballroom circuit repels them and deters them from learning to dance at all, as the glittery and glamorous image becomes their only mental picture of social dance. For our purposes in this book, it is most important that you know that this end of the spectrum of formality exists, but it is not reality for most of the social dancers out there. If it is your personal dancing goal, budget accordingly, and this book will get you started with a firm foundation in the basics. If the glitz is not for you, keep reading, because there is much more to the world of dance.

Informal

At the opposite end of the spectrum from the glamorous world of ballroom competition and performance, you will find the informal venues for social dance. This is where the majority of people find enormous satisfaction from their acquired social dance skills. You do not need fancy costumes, expensive shoes, or even a hardwood floor to dance socially. All you need is some good music that gets you moving (or the ability to hum or whistle a tune) and a dance partner.

Many an evening in has been spent dancing in the living room or on the back patio to favorite songs. If you have the luxury and the energy to make an evening out, you can dance socially at many venues, from a restaurant with some tables pushed aside to a country-western nightclub where denim is the most prevalent fabric in the room.

Interestingly enough, you can see and practice several couples dances in either of these settings in casual attire and a relaxed atmosphere. Sometimes you don't even need music to practice your dancing; a beautiful sunset at a beach is inspiration enough. You and your partner can slow dance to the rhythm of the waves crashing on the shore and christen dusk with a final dip as the sun sets on the water.

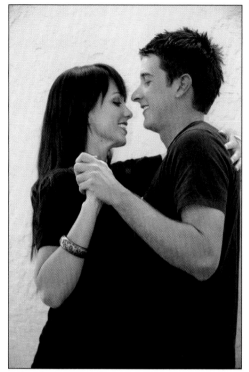

© **istockphoto.com/Renee Lee**

Social Dancing Subcultures

SOCIAL DANCING can be divided into four main subcultures, although other microcosms exist. The four main subcultures consist of ballroom, country, swing, and Latin, even though they're all still under the umbrella of social dancing. As you will see, there is overlap between the actual dances practiced in each category; for example, the cha-cha is done in ballroom, country-western, and Latin styles of couples dance, but the subculture, music, and the finer points of styling differ between each of the categories.

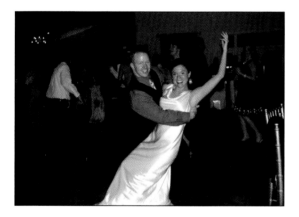

Ballroom

Ballroom encompasses the traditional world of couples dance instruction and practice. Dance legends Arthur Murray and Fred Astaire are the champions and shapers of this subculture. "Traditional" is the word that defines ballroom subculture. The music is traditional, the dances are traditional, and the instruction is highly structured and standardized across the country and around the world. Money also comes to mind in the ballroom culture.

Where to Learn and Attire for Learning

One goes to a ballroom or a dance studio to learn the ballroom style of couples dancing. At these studios you will find standardized curriculums published by centralized governing dance associations. The various teachers at each of the studios certify at different levels just like the students, so at a glance you should be able to see what a teacher is qualified to teach. Because the ballroom subculture is the most formal of the social dance styles, attire for lessons is slightly more formal than for the other styles. Although any studio or ballroom would recommend you be comfortable as you learn to dance, baggy sweatpants and grubby sneakers are not the most appropriate attire for a ballroom dance lesson. Business-casual clothing with comfortable close-heeled shoes (no flip-flops or sandals) is appropriate if you are just starting. If you decide that DanceSport is your passion, you can invest at a later date in specialized dance athletic apparel and ballroom shoes.

Where to Dance and Attire for Going out Dancing

Believe it or not, a ballroom is one of the most common places to go out and practice your dancing. Ballrooms host various dances in the evening during the week and occasionally on the weekends. Different evenings have different themes, so most studios and ballrooms publish a monthly calendar that you can use to plan your social schedule accordingly. You can also dance to ballroom-style music at weddings and other formal special events.

It is completely appropriate and even recommended to dress to the nines to go to an evening dance at a ballroom. Ladies, pull out your sequined shirts, fancy skirts, hose, and fancy shoes if you don't have specialty suede or leather-soled ballroom dance shoes. Gentlemen, shirt-and-tie combinations or "going-out" shirts with slacks and polished shoes (again, ballroom dance shoes are recommended but not necessary) are within the dress code for a ballroom social dance event.

Most Popular Dances

Ballroom is the most structured of the styles of social dancing, with regimented competitions and clear-cut syllabi for instruction. The dances that you would typically see and learn in a ballroom include the waltz, foxtrot, quickstep, swing, cha-cha, rumba, salsa, and tango.

Of Special Note

As you decide which style of social dancing is right for you, please bear in mind budget and lesson schedules. Ballroom instruction is unique in that most of the lessons take place Monday through Friday during bankers' hours. Almost all ballrooms offer group classes and some private lessons in the evenings, but the majority of their instruction is during regular business hours.

Country

Country is the all-American apple pie answer to social dancing. The music is country-western, the feel is casual and the least stylized of the four subcultures, and denim is acceptable on almost every occasion. Cowboy hats and boots come to mind when country social dancing is mentioned; although they are not required for casual social dancing, they are prevalent and appropriate. Depending on what part of the country you are in, you might need to wear sunglasses to protect your eyes from the glare off of the well-polished belt buckles.

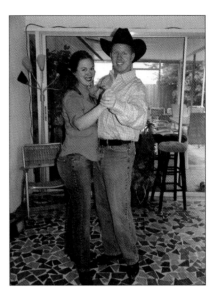

Where to Learn and Attire for Learning

One can learn country dances at some of the local dance studios, but your best bet for getting started in your local area with country social dancing are your local country bars and nightclubs. Here you can learn the basics of the various country social dances and meet the instructors. Most of the instructors on the country circuit are freelance teachers who teach at the nightclubs in the early evenings and teach private lessons during the week and on weekends. Be comfortable and wear jeans when you go to learn country social dancing. You would most likely feel slightly overdressed if you wore the same outfit you selected for a ballroom lesson to a country bar for a beginner two-step lesson. If you have cowboy boots, wear them—they help you get into the feel of the music and culture. Ladies, close-heeled shoes are appropriate when learning social dancing in any of the subcultures. *Never wear flip-flops or open-heeled sandals or mules to a couples social dance lesson.* If you forget this rule, chances are you will only forget it once. Close-toed shoes are also recommended for ladies, especially while your dance partner gets the hang of the basic steps and leading.

Where to Dance and Attire for Going out Dancing

Country nightclubs and bars are the best places to go out dancing in the country social dance subculture. Most large country nightclubs make it a point to have a large, well-maintained hardwood dance floor with convenient rails on which to set drinks and lean surrounding the floor. Ladies, if you want to wear a skirt or a dress you can, but chances are you will feel overdressed. A sparkly or fun top with jeans (at any age) and close-toed, close-heeled shoes are appropriate attire for a lady at a country nightclub. Likewise, gentlemen, don't even bother with anything dry-clean only. Jeans and a clean-collared shirt are appropriate, with either cowboy boots or non-sneaker shoes. Casual is key.

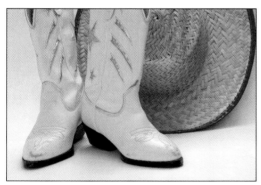

© istockphoto.com/Ronda Oliver

Most Popular Dances

You might be surprised at the variety of dances you will see in the country subculture. On any given evening in a country nightclub, you can see and dance with people doing the two-step, triple two-step, waltz, cha-cha, slow dance, swing, West coast swing, polka, and even occasionally the hustle. In addition to the couples dancing, there is also a lot of attention to line dancing, which is done by individuals. You might also want to give a few dances a try and head to a lesson to get your feet wet with it as well.

Of Special Note

If you are budget-conscious with your entertainment discretionary spending, country might be the initial route for you to take. Group lessons are extremely inexpensive, private lessons are usually significantly less expensive than in a ballroom, the appropriate attire is most likely already hanging in your closet or sitting in your drawer, and cover charges at country nightclubs are usually negligible when compared to other dance venues. Also, if you are interested in learning to couples dance but you're afraid of looking or feeling frou-frou or effeminate, the country scene and the country style of social dancing are as no-frills as they come. For many people, the country subculture eases the transition into the world of couples dance, regardless of whether they are huge fans of country music.

Swing

Swing encompasses the family of dances that were born from the jazz and big-band eras. Swing dance subculture is a movement in the dance community that has gained enormous popularity since the mid 1990s and has supported a resurgence of "retro" clothing, music, and dance.

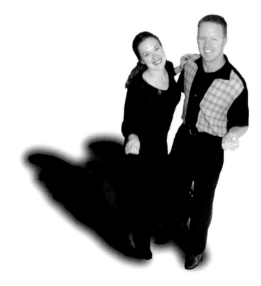

Where to Learn and Attire for Learning

You can learn some version of swing at any ball-room or dance studio. However, to find group lessons and get your foot in your local swing dance community, your best bet would probably be to go online. Many of the swing dance clubs around the country are created and populated by computer-savvy people in their twenties and thirties, although at a swing dance you will probably see all age groups, from high school up through senior citizens. Swing dancing in a ballroom and swing dancing at a swing dance have entirely different looks and feels. Swing dances are often held weekly and/or monthly, but swing nightclubs are not prevalent in all parts of the country—often the swing club or group will rent out a given facility for the lessons and event. Be comfortable if you are going to a swing dance lesson. You do not need to be as formal as you would be for a ballroom lesson, but denim is not recommended. Business-casual dress with comfortable close-heeled shoes is recommended for both ladies and gentlemen for a swing lesson.

Where to Dance and Attire for Going out Dancing

As mentioned in the previous section, not every city or geographical area has a venue specifically dedicated to swing dancing like they do for the other three subcultures. A search for your local city and swing dance should reveal a local swing dance group or two. Because swing dances are not always held in nightclubs, it is unique to swing dance and ballroom dance that their events are often non-smoking. When dressing for an evening out swing dancing, you have a couple of options. You can go with business-casual attire for the ladies and gentle-men, and just look nice and clean-cut, or if you have them on hand, you can go all out and go vintage. Many swing dance aficionados have fairly elaborate vintage wardrobes to truly step back into the big-band era. As always, close-heeled shoes are a must.

Most Popular Dances

The swing subculture includes the lindy hop, jitter-bug, jive, East coast swing, balboa, and West coast swing. You will find, however, that most swing dancers only truly dance one or two of the swing dances and simply know what the others are.

Of Special Note

Swing dance is probably the least intimidating form of social dancing to get your feet wet with. However, depending on your geographical area, it can be a little difficult to find swing dance venues. If you are interested in swing but you can't seem to get wind of your local swing events, try country. Many of the instructors cross over between the swing and country subcultures and can probably point you in the right direction.

Latin

Latin couples dancing is the hot and spicy corner of the dance world. Just as the dances and subcultures vary in different parts of Latin America, so the Latin dances and related dance subcultures vary across the globe.

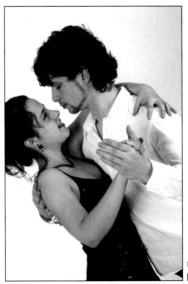

© istockphoto.com/
Paul Piebinga

Where to Learn and Attire for Learning

You can find Latin dance instruction at many ball-rooms; however, once you have the hang of the basic timing and some of the foundational moves, you might want to broaden your horizons. If you want to learn the truly Latin versions of the dances and dance in the subculture, you might be better off seeking out a specialized dance studio or a free-lance instructor who teaches salsa, meringue, bacchata, or cha-cha at a local Latin nightclub or even restaurant. The dress code might be dictated by where you are learning to dance and whether you will be staying out dancing to practice following your lesson. That being said, you should strive to be comfortable when learning the Latin dances; you will be getting an aerobic workout, especially with salsa. When learning, wear as comfortable of shoes as possible. Save your feet for when you go out dancing.

Where to Dance and Attire for Going out Dancing

Salsa clubs are the most popular place to go out Latin dancing. Prepare yourself for a high-energy evening followed by a day of very sore feet. When Latin dancers, particularly salsa dancers, show up to party, they get down to business and go until the wee hours of the morning. Be prepared to dress to the nines in your club wear—ladies, this is the only dance subculture where strappy sandals are not only acceptable, but the norm for footwear. A few words of caution for the ladies regarding footwear: Try not to twist or break your ankles, and try to protect your toes from errant feet of other dancers. Gentlemen, dress sharply and wear polished shoes. Your clothing will most likely be dictated by your local climate and the season for both ladies and gentlemen.

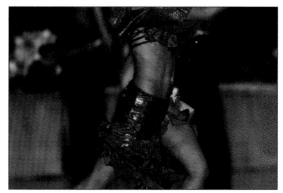
© istockphoto.com/Roberto Adrian

Most Popular Dances

The most popular Latin dance is the salsa. There are several types of salsa out there, some of them being "called" dances, similar to a square dance, except they are performed in a circle (no corners necessary). However, the rumba, tango, meringue, bacchata, cha-cha, mambo, and samba also fall into the Latin dance category.

Of Special Note

As you dive into the Latin dancing subculture, keep in mind two key descriptive terms: fun and sensual. The Latin dances are often described as the most fun and sensual of all four social dance subcultures. As with any of the dance subcultures, it is important to be sensitive to cultural differences as you get out and embark upon new communities of people—everyone is out dancing to have a good time. If you are not Latin American by birth or heritage, keep in mind that you are immersing yourself in a corner of someone else's heritage for the evening, so be respectful of that.

Dance Instruction Types

BEFORE JUMPING right in and taking dance lessons, you might want to consider taking a few minutes and reading this next section. Much like everything that's been talked about in the book so far, there are many different ways of learning and many different situations where it can take place. There are three main ways that people learn couples dancing:

► **Private lessons**

► **Group lessons**

► **DIY (Do It Yourself)**

Everyone is different, so it's hard to say that any one way is better than the others. With that in mind, we'll just break them down and talk a little bit about each one.

Private Lessons

Private lessons usually consist of one or two students and one instructor. The private setting allows you to get tailored instruction to fit your dance styles, habits, or shortcomings. You can learn to dance in a relatively short period of time with private lessons if your budget will allow it. Private lessons are common in ballroom dance studios and normally run anywhere from about $45 to $150 per hour. You can also find freelance instructors in your area who often have an hourly rate that is less expensive than a local ballroom. Most people take private lessons so they can learn at their own pace and not have to worry about dancing in front of others. Some people take private lessons strictly to have a partner to dance with in a social setting, while others do it for the health benefits, in the same way that people hire personal trainers at a gym to walk them through their daily workouts. Whatever the reason, private lessons can be extremely beneficial if you end up with the right instructor.

Group Lessons

Group lessons usually consist of one or two instructors and anywhere from about six to a hundred people. In group dance lessons there is no standard for minimum or maximum class size. The group setting differs from the private setting in that the information is general and not specifically tailored to your dancing as an individual. Even if you're taking private lessons, group lessons can reinforce your learning without too much of a budget constraint. Group lessons are more affordable than private lessons and can run anywhere from about $3 per class to $25 per class, and usually there are no contracts involved. There are many social benefits of going to group classes, including meeting other people interested in social dancing, getting a chance to dance and practice with a number of partners throughout your evening, not being the center of attention or having an instructor watching every move you make, and having the ability to watch and learn from the others in the class. In addition to the social benefits, going to different group classes also gives you a chance to see, meet, and evaluate a few instructors in your area.

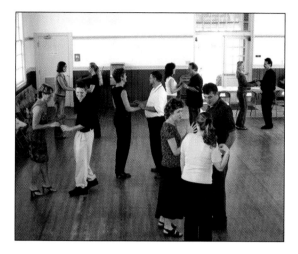

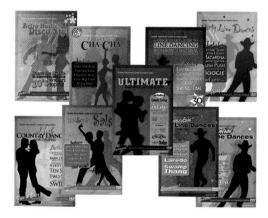

DIY (Do It Yourself)

A third and increasingly more common approach to learning to dance is through self-teaching. Though some of the social benefits are not present with learning by a book, video, or DVD, there are many other benefits that can be derived. First and foremost, you'll get structure and documentation when you do it on your own. Second, you'll be able to learn on your own time and set your own schedule. Third, you'll be able to visualize and conceptualize the dancing as you go by looking at pictures or video of what you're learning. When you first start out in dancing, you'll be creating what's called *muscle memory*.

> **Muscle memory** describes the process by which certain physical movements, such as dance steps, become automatic. Once you have established a step in your muscle memory, you no longer have to think about it while you execute it—it becomes natural to your body.

For learning or reinforcing the basics the right way to pave a road for future learning, it's best to have some type of reference material to go back to that has the exact information you'll need on it. Learning on your own is much more affordable and less time-constrained than learning in either group lessons or private lessons, but it is best to use it as one type of instruction and not the only one. Supplement either private or group lessons with the book-and-DVD combination, and you'll be surprised at how quickly you feel confident in the dance world.

Choosing Your Instructor

In the final chapter, "Picture Yourself Dancing for Life," you'll find detailed information on next steps for all your dances and for choosing an instructor to assist you with the more intermediate and advanced levels of dancing. There are specific qualities and attributes for several different situations that you should be aware of when seeking out further instruction. Once you're comfortable with the basics of each of the dances, or the ones that you really want to know, you'll feel much more confident in going out, watching, and talking with instructors in your area. When you're ready to progress past the basics, you'll find this section to be invaluable because it will help you determine what's best for you.

Rhythm and Music for Beginning Dancers

CONTRARY TO POPULAR BELIEF, you do not need to know much about music to be a great dancer. Assuming you know very little about music, we're going to get you started here with the essentials that will have you feeling like a pro in no time. We'll briefly describe what you need to know about each of the following terms, and then we'll talk about how to apply these concepts to dance.

▶ **Beat.** The heartbeat of the music. What you would tap your feet to. The recurring pulsation that is constant and regular. Watch a metronome or a second hand on a clock or a watch, and you'll understand what to relate the beat to.

▶ **Step/count.** The amount of time allocated to each step taken. For example, a "slow" step denotes a step requiring two beats of music, and a "quick" step denotes a step requiring only one beat of music.

▶ **Measure.** The number of beats grouped together according to the time signature (the top number). For example, in most songs you'll hear a series of eight beats that continue to repeat themselves through the entire song.

▶ **Downbeat.** The first beat of a given measure. This is your starting point. You first have to know when the measure is ready to repeat itself, and then you get ready and go so that your first step is actually down on the first beat, or downbeat. This is where the expression "5-6-7-8" becomes extremely useful, because it prepares you for the ending of a measure and gives you your starting point.

▶ **Upbeat.** The last beat of a given measure. This beat is often called an "and" count when starting to move with the music. Rather than the "5-6-7-8" mentioned in the previous bullet point, one might say "ready, and" and then start dancing. It would be the equivalent of the count 8 in the previous example.

▶ **Rhythm.** The arrangement of beats in a given song. Essentially, rhythm is symmetrical groupings formed by the regular recurrence of either heavy or light accents. In a regular rhythm, the dancer's movements should look natural and be even and symmetrical, and all walking steps should be the same length.

▶ **Tempo.** The rate of "speed" of the music, measured in BPM (*beats per minute*). This is how you determine whether the song is slow, medium, or fast, and it will give you an idea of what dance to dance.

▶ **Phrase.** Two or more measures grouped together. This is more important for advanced dancers in dealing with choreography or in social dancing when you are trying to align your dance with the structure of the song, but it's good to understand. It may or may not help you immediately, but it will one day prove its value.

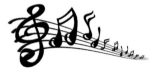

© istockphoto.com/Steven Bourelle

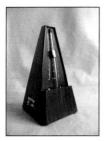

Practice what you just learned by trying the following steps. First set the stage by using either a metronome or some kind of device that keeps a steady beat aloud so you'll be able to follow along with it. Set the speed to go about one beat per second. This will give you approximately 60 BPM, or a tempo of 60 to start the following steps:

1. Count the beats aloud in a repeating eight-beat fashion. Start with one, go all the way through eight, and then start over with one, and so on. This will get you more familiar with what a measure is.

2. Clap your hands to the beat of the music, then snap your fingers to the beat of the music, and then tap either foot to the beat of the music. Do each one at least eight times to get a decent amount of practice.

3. Identify the upbeat and the downbeat and try to take a step each time the downbeat occurs. It doesn't matter which foot; you're simply trying to align your perception with your motor skills. The upbeat is where you'd start your motion, and the downbeat is where you'd come down to the floor with your foot.

4. Try walking with "slow" steps, which take up two beats. Start on the downbeat, or one, and walk on the numbers one, three, five, and seven, and then repeat it over and over. You can do this in place, in a small circle, or however it best fits in the room. The idea on this one is to take a step and then hold a beat, and then continue. Try not to completely stop while you're holding the beat, though—it will look choppy and unnatural.

5. Try walking with "quick" steps, which take up only one beat each. Start on the downbeat, or one, and walk on the numbers one, two, three, four, five, six, seven, and eight, and then repeat it over and over. Just like in Step 4, you can do it in whatever fashion best suits your surroundings.

6. Try walking with a combination of "slow" steps and "quick" steps. Start with doing eight slows and eight quicks, then try it with four slows and four quicks, and then try it by doing just two slows then two quicks, and repeat it over and over again.

The combination of the two slows and two quicks is very common in all types of social dancing and is something you really should spend some time working on before you get too far along. If you're able to transition between the two and feel as though you're doing so smoothly and evenly, then your rhythm is also being strengthened. If you don't feel natural yet, try to relax and take a deep breath. Dancing is nothing more than walking to different speeds, so if your walk is natural, it's just a matter of time until you can incorporate it into your dancing.

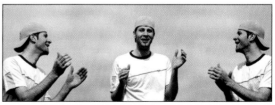

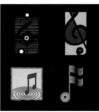

Leading and Following versus Choreography

"THEY'RE SO BEAUTIFUL together out on the dance floor. They must have had their dance choreographed!" Did they? Maybe. What exactly is choreography, and how is it different than lead-and-follow dancing? Well, each dance is a compilation of various moves that can be matched and mismatched throughout a song to produce the end-product dance. Choreography is when these moves are arranged in a predetermined pattern and are performed the same way with each repetition. Lead-and-follow dancing differs from choreography in the freedom of arrangement of the moves within a dance. A choreographed dance and a lead-and-follow dance can both have the same 15 moves used three times apiece. In the choreographed dance, you would end up with the same choreographed routine repeated three times, but in the lead-and-follow routine, you would see a dance with no discernable repetition.

Is it possible to have a beautiful, flowing dance without choreography? Absolutely. Lead-and-follow

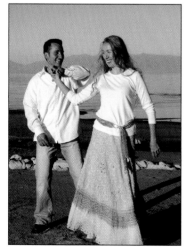

dancing can be just as elegant as choreographed dancing if both partners clearly understand the basic steps of the dance and their individual roles in their partnership on the dance floor.

© istockphoto.com/Renee Lee

Social dancing parallels other sports in more than just cardiovascular and physiological benefits for the participants. Lead-and-follow relationships exist in other corners of the sporting world in addition to the dance floor of a ballroom. For instance, imagine an all-American football game—the stands are packed with excited spectators, and the energy from the field is palpable. An intricate lead-and-follow plotline is about to unfold as the ball is kicked off.

Leading would be the equivalent of the quarterback calling each play at the line of scrimmage based on the situation (the players, the defense, the time clock, and so on). Following would be what the rest of the offense would do based on what the quarterback called. When the play is over, the quarterback reassesses the field and game situation and calls another play, and the game continues with the quarterback leading the offense through a selection of plays based on the score, field position, player composition, weather, and so on.

Choreography would be the equivalent of the entire offense putting a collection of plays together in a very specific order and calling it something like "First Quarter Plays." With choreography, when the offense takes the field, they know exactly what they're going to do on the first play, on the second play, on the third, and so on, regardless of the situation or who they're playing. If someone is injured, the play continues on, just less that player and their role in the play sequence.

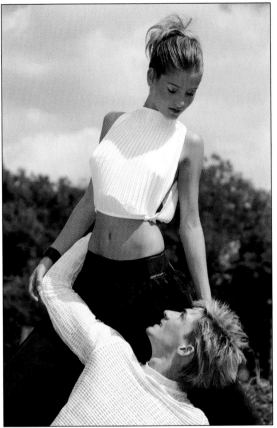

© istockphoto.com/Maciej Laska

Lead-and-follow dancing combines a number of skills that are tested on every dance outing and in every dance. The skills that must be mastered include the dance floor basics (covered in Chapter 2), a clear understanding of both the leaders' and the followers' responsibilities, the basics of whatever dance you're dancing, and a great deal of common courtesy and respect toward others. Though leading and following might appear a bit overwhelming, the pieces that make up the whole are not overly complicated by themselves and can be picked up with just a little practice.

Although good choreography and seamless lead-and-follow dancing are indistinguishable to the untrained observer, choreography often deviates from the basics of social dance because it is a learned pattern in which both parties know the entire sequence of movements in advance rather than depending on interpersonal communication on the dance floor to create the dance on the spot. In a choreographed dance, both partners are taught the exact steps and the order in which they'll dance them.

Although both choreography and lead-and-follow dancing involve tremendous amounts of practice and commitment, there are definite differences between the two. The main difference between leading and following and choreography is that one is for dancing with others in social situations (leading and following) and the other is for dancing a routine with a specific individual, either for a special event, such as a wedding, or in a competition. Typically, a choreographed routine is useable only with a specific partner and only really looks good with the song for which the dance was choreographed. Understanding the fundamentals of social dancing, including footwork and floor position, as well as the basics of partner dancing is critical in both types of dancing.

The advantages of this type of dancing are that both partners know what's coming up and know exactly where they need to be. Some people need and like this kind of structure, and it works great for them. People who are getting married often want a short choreographed routine to do to their first dance because neither partner wants to take a chance leading or following in front of others. The disadvantage of a choreographed dance is that it's usually a dance that can only be done with the partner you learned it with, and oftentimes it's to a specific song. There are typically very few lead-and-follow elements to a choreographed dance, yet they are made to look the part.

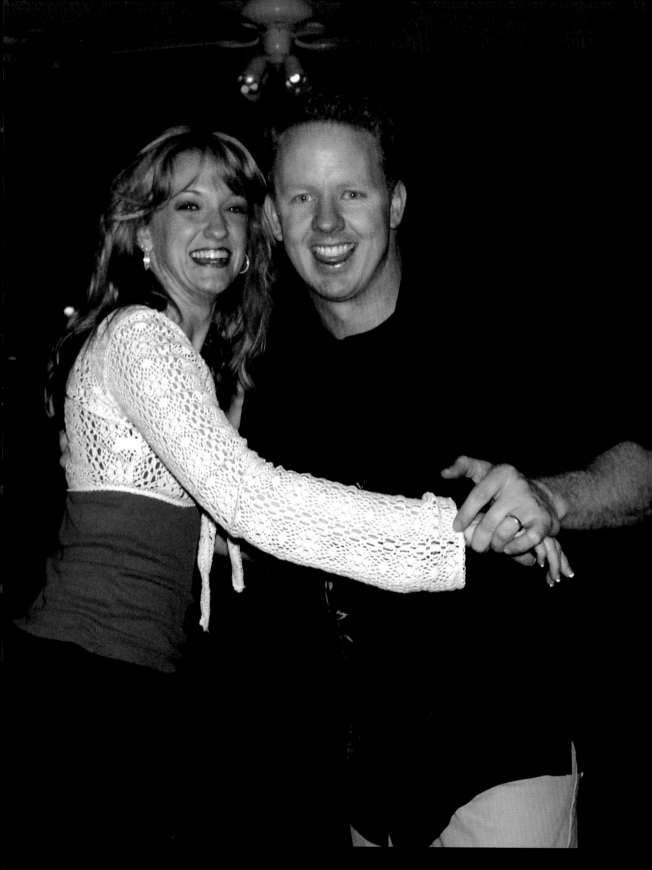

2

Beginner *Basics*

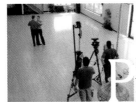

PICTURE YOURSELF stepping confidently onto the dance floor, cocking your head to the side to listen to the music for a moment, and then transitioning smoothly into the line of dance—on beat, with the right foot, and matching your partner perfectly. If you are having difficulty picturing this as your reality, read on. In this chapter, you will fill your toolbox with the essentials needed to construct the nine dances taught in the remaining chapters of this book. You will learn the three rules by which to live and learn, four connection points, and five foot positions. You will then build your knowledge base by adding the six basic dance positions, seven essential steps, and eight directional possibilities. Once you have mastered those nuts and bolts, you will learn the essentials of leading and following—the principles that are universal to all of the social dances—and get warmed up and ready to dive in and learn your first social dance. From the how-to's of dancing with a partner to mastering such concepts as perception-motor match, this chapter will start you out on the proverbial "right foot."

Dance Etiquette for Any Situation

BOTH PARTNER ETIQUETTE and floor etiquette are emphasized throughout this book. Following are some specifics on both partner etiquette and floor etiquette.

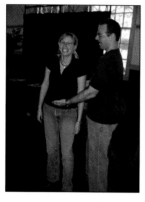

Partner Etiquette

When you are dancing, the two most important people on the dance floor are yourself and your dance partner. The following rules will make your joint dancing experience, especially during the learning period, much more enjoyable.

Do Not Give Unsolicited Advice

Unsolicited advice is arsenic to your newly formed dance partnership. In the great big world outside of the realm of dance, know-it-alls are unwelcome, and on the dance floor the same rule applies. Leave your "I'm an expert" hat at home when you come to learn how to dance. The only exclusion to this rule is when you are the paid instructor. By paying the fee and attending the class, the student(s) have waived their rights to give unsolicited advice. They have designated the instructor as the expert, and it is then the instructor's job to give advice and correct problems as he or she sees them—with tact and aplomb on every occasion.

Trust Your Partner

Always trust that your partner will do the correct action as soon as he or she possibly can. At least eight times out of ten, if your partner is not executing a step or move correctly, it is because his or her arms or legs aren't quite getting the message from the brain yet, not because your partner didn't understand the move. Social dance was created as a leisure activity, and by nature should be pleasurable to the participants. Though the intentions are usually pure, the results are often disastrous when beginning dancers violate rules one and two of partner etiquette. Remembering the old adage about removing the log from your own eye prior to pointing out the splinter in your dance partner's can salvage a difficult dance session.

Thank Your Partner

Miss Manners would be proud if all dancers remembered this simple rule. Please be polite on the social dance floor and thank your partner for the dance. Even if it is through gritted teeth due to painful smashed toes, a simple "Thank you for the dance" goes a long way.

Always Introduce Yourself

This final rule of partner dance etiquette is probably the most frequently overlooked in the social dance world. People attend dances and go out to nightclubs in order to dance and meet other people, but they often forget the simple step of introducing themselves to a new dance partner in their zeal to show off their spiffy moves. Remember, dancing is a social event, and it is socially astute to at least learn someone's name before invading his or her personal space by assuming dance position!

Floor Etiquette

An essential yet often overlooked aspect of successful social dancing is floor etiquette. Dancing on a social dance floor is much like driving. Often new drivers learn in an empty parking lot or some other controlled environment. They gain confidence in their own skills and ability to maneuver their car, only to discover the difficult part of driving once you master the basics is not pointing your own car in the direction you want to go and hitting the gas; rather, it is negotiating all of the hazards along the way (otherwise known as traffic). In the same way, a beginning dancer can be thrown for a loop after mastering the basic steps for the two-step, only to discover that negotiating a crowded dance floor in a country nightclub for an upbeat two-step is much akin to merging into traffic on the beltway around Boston, Massachusetts—traffic is bumper to bumper, with everyone going at least fifty-five miles per hour! The following three rules should significantly improve your chances for success and enjoyment on the social dance floor.

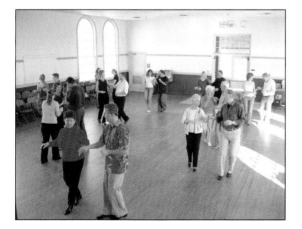

Be Aware of Your Surroundings

On a crowded dance floor your surroundings are always changing. In the interest of preventing collisions and other unhappy events, awareness of the layout of the floor and all obstacles, moving and otherwise, is necessary. This responsibility falls primarily on the leader because he is in charge of selecting the moves, and in dances that move around the circumference of the floor, the leader is usually in the forward-facing position while the follower spends most of her time moving backward around the floor. That being said, it is also important for the follower to be aware of her surroundings. There are some collisions that only the follower can see coming, so if you can see over your partner's shoulder, followers, pay attention and alert your leader if you see anything!

Apologize or Excuse Yourself

If a collision occurs on the dance floor, always apologize or excuse yourself, even if the other person ran into you. Think of it this way—you are either apologizing for running into someone, or you are apologizing for not seeing the other dancer's disastrous course and taking the high road of collision prevention. Even if you don't feel that the collision was your fault, apologize in the interest of a pleasant evening. Engaging another dancer's ego in a contest to determine whose fault a collision really was is rarely in anyone's best interest. Save any disparaging remarks for a pillow or other inanimate and non-emotive object.

Know the Correct Placement for Each Dance

Collision prevention is even more effective in the battle against spoiled evenings of dance than collision management. The first step of collision prevention is knowledge of the dance and the correct placement of that dance on the dance floor. For instance, to dance the two-step, waltz, or tango successfully, it is vitally important to know that these dances are danced around the circumference of the dance floor with constant movement in the counterclockwise direction.

Two Rules of the Road

THERE ARE TWO MAJOR RULES in couples dancing that every dancer must have tattooed in his or her memory.

1. Ladies are *always* right.

2. Men *always* get what is left.

Ladies Are Always Right

The lady's first step in every dance will always be taken with her right foot. Hence, ladies are always right. It is not clear why this was initially established, but it has been opined that the original inventors of the rules of dance decided that the ladies were always right to compensate for the fact that the men were the designated leaders of the dances. The rules of leading and following will be discussed at further length later in this chapter, but in the meantime, let it suffice that ladies are always right.

From this point forward, this text will be using the terms woman, women, lady, ladies, and follower interchangeably. Although it is not necessary for the leader to be a man and the follower to be a woman, these are the traditional roles, and the instruction on the DVD (as well as standard ballroom and studio instruction) uses the same terminology. Conversely, the leaders will be referred to as men, gentlemen, and leaders interchangeably.

As mentioned previously, this means that the first step of every dance for the follower, or lady, will be taken with her right foot. Consequently, the follower needs to become accustomed to waiting in ready position, with her weight on her left foot, ready to take the first step with the right.

Men Always Get What's Left

Speaking of the men, those of you who are learning the leader's part of the dances need to remember that men always get what is left. This means that you will always start a dance with your left foot. So, when you are waiting in a ready position for a dance to start, you will be standing with your weight on your right foot, ready to take that first step with the left.

The practical aspect of these two rules is geared toward the prevention of toe-smashing. This is easily demonstrated if you and your dance partner stand facing each other, about 12 inches apart. Both men and women stand in your ready position, as just described. On the count of three, men will take one step forward and ladies will take one step backward. One, two, three.... Were you successful in toe-smashing avoidance? Hopefully you ended up with the man having his left foot in front of his right and the lady with her right foot behind her left. Had you both stepped with your right or both stepped with your left, the lady's toes most likely would have been crushed, and that would have been the end of that lesson or evening out!

Remember—ladies are always right, and men always get what's left.

Three Rules for Life, Learning, and Dance

THREE CONCEPTS govern all the rules of etiquette that will impact your ability to learn and practice social dancing. The mastery of these concepts will dramatically increase your success rate in the "classroom"—referring to wherever you are learning, be it a ballroom or your living room—as well as on the dance floor, once you are out practicing and enjoying your new skills. These three concepts are ones to keep in the back of your mind even after you have put this book up on the shelf and mastered all of the dance moves and steps taught in these pages. These three bits of wisdom to remember are respect for self, respect for others, and responsibility for all of your actions.

Respect for Self

When you show "respect for self," you enable yourself to learn to dance as well as learn to dance with a partner. As you show respect for your body, you will treat it accordingly. Posture improves, carriage improves, and you begin to look like a dancer. A person who respects his or her body holds the head up and the shoulders back. This person also respects the limitations of his or her body. When you dance, you also need to show respect for your intelligence and ability to learn. When you are confident in your own mind's ability to learn the material, you will learn it faster.

Respect for Others

Because social dancing involves more than one person by definition, showing respect for others is imperative. This includes respecting their bodies, physical limitations, learning styles, and learning paces. Most of all, respect your dance partner's personal space. If he or she looks uncomfortable in the particular position you are learning, exercise your communication skills and fix the problem as best you can. If your dance partner has a particular limitation that physically won't allow him or her to do a particular movement, talk about it and move on. As mentioned earlier, social dancing is multidimensional, and most moves are optional in a dance. Change to a move that may be a challenge, but also a possibility, and don't get discouraged. Respect your partner's learning style and pace. If your partner needs to watch the DVD to truly grasp a concept visually, don't rush through it and get frustrated when he or she doesn't execute the move properly prior to viewing the DVD.

Responsibility for All of Your Actions

The third and final rule to live and learn to dance by is to take responsibility for all of your actions. The blame game is a pursuit of frustration that can only end in disaster for your dancing career and sometimes your relationship. Once you take responsibility for a mistake, you can take the next step and figure out how to fix the problem and prevent repetition of the incorrect movement. This will expedite your learning process and prevent the formation of "bad" muscle memory. As you take responsibility for your actions, it will encourage your dance partner to take responsibility for his or her own mistakes and will re-center the focus on the problems and the dance, rather than on each other. When you are responsible for your mistakes, you are also responsible for your successes.

The Four Basic Connection Points

A DANCE FRAME is much like a picture frame in that it is meant to hold the subject in a position that allows for optimal viewing. Creating the perfect dance frame is quite elementary and can be done without ever having danced a single step. The key ingredients are two people and a general conceptual understanding of four connection points.

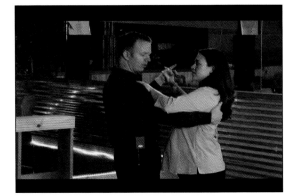

Here you'll find the four basic connection points that will enable you to create your frame. Once you are able to go through each one and understand them without question, you'll find yourself getting in and out of frame just for fun to practice and build muscle memory. It is important to note that creating your dance frame while you are relaxed and stationary is a much different experience from maintaining the dance frame throughout a dance. You will find that a dance frame is easily created while standing in place, yet in motion, such as in dancing, the frame must be continuously adjusted to account for different dance positions, sudden weight changes, reductions in the number of connection points, or any number of other situations.

In subsequent chapters you will see how to incorporate the different connection points into each dance and when and how to change them to create a new look.

It's time to start the hands-on portion of your learning experience. Literally—you and your dance partner are going to build your dance frame one connection point at a time. To do this, it is best to stand facing your partner with your feet about shoulder-width apart, with somewhere between one-and-a-half and three feet between the two of you. Check to make sure that you have soft knees. Try to smile and, most importantly, don't forget to breathe!

Soft knees are created by standing with your legs almost straight, knees just slightly bent. You rarely want to fully straighten your legs when dancing because this "locks out" your knees and prevents you from easily changing weight from foot to foot or from moving smoothly. Soft knees allows for optimal circulation in your legs, as well as legs that are ready to move in any direction at a moment's notice.

Connection Point One

To establish connection point 1, the leader's left hand and the follower's right hand should be held up at the shorter person's shoulder level, as though you were both waving a casual hello. The leader then shifts the angle of his hand so the fingers are pointing to his upper left rather than straight up in the air. The follower's hand can then meet his, palm to palm, and she can gently close her fingers down between his thumb and fingers. Both partners can then close all of the fingers—*gently*. It is important to note that the important part of this connection point is the pressure between the two palms, *not* the clasping of the two hands.

Connection points are made by creating tension at particular places where dance partners' bodies meet. This tension allows for nonverbal communication of direction changes, foot movements, and other dance moves. These communications between the partners are known as *leads*.

In other words, you technically could create connection point 1 by simply pressing your palms together—the closing of your fingers and thumbs is simply for looks. Refer to the picture on the right to check your position. Make sure your connection point 1 is right in the middle of the space between the two of you, so that neither partner has to overextend to make this connection point work. Each partner should be pushing slightly toward the other partner through the palm of his or her hand. It is imperative that each partner hold his or her own hand up and, most importantly, that neither partner squeezes the other's hand. If your partner is putting too much pressure on your hand or

squeezing it at all, please let him or her know before you get any further. If you don't want to say anything, just squeeze back a time or two in nice, quick, repetitive motions to let your partner know. Make sure your eyes are watching your hand when you do it, then look back at your partner and smile. Chances are your partner will know what you were doing. Ensure that connection point 1 does not go above the shorter person's shoulder so as to enable optimal visibility for the dancer as well as onlookers, and especially if there are going to be any pictures taken during the dance.

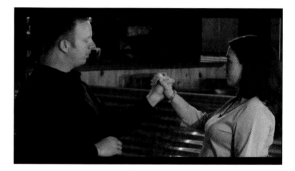

Connection Point Two

Go ahead and release your arms from connection point 1 for a moment and shake them out. If you hold the dance frame for a long period of time before your arm and back muscles have adjusted to the new position, you will feel like your arms are going to fall off. Although you released connection point 1, remain in the same foot and body positions you were in so you can create connection point 2.

Connection point 1 is not needed for connection point 2 to take place.

The second connection point involves the leader's right palm, or hand, and the follower's left shoulder blade—or scapula, for the more technical term. Leaders, you'll take your right palm and place it across the follower's shoulder blade. Ladies, it is best if you lift your left arm up and out of the way—just don't rest it on top of the leader's arm yet. Now, ladies, you want to make sure you're leaning slightly back and that you're being fully supported by that hand. If it's done correctly, you should be able to try to fall backward (not straight down) and not be able to because of the connection between the leader's right hand and your shoulder blade.

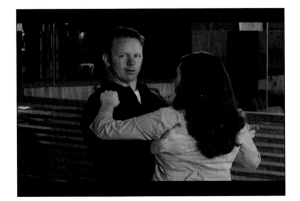

Leaders, your partner's shoulder blade should be right in the middle of your hand and you should be able to pull slightly with your fingers to the right to get your partner to move to your right or push slightly with the palm of your hand toward the left to get your partner to move to your left.

Pushing and pulling could also be described as *guiding*. A slight push or pull should be the equivalent of a smooth guide in practice.

Connection point 2 should be practiced by the leader attempting to move the follower to the right, to the left, forward, and backward, solely based on connection point 2. Practice these motions slowly and make sure both partners are perfectly clear on the directions. Followers, make sure you're not thinking about what's happening and that you're letting your body weight fall into the hand of your partner. Leaders, make sure your movements are clear and confident. The follower should not have to think about where to go; she should be guided smoothly in any single direction.

Another good way to practice is for both partners to go through the exercise of moving in different directions with their eyes closed. Next, try it with just the follower's eyes closed—then, just the leader's. Practice this exercise until you're both comfortable with the motion and concept.

Connection point 2 is critical because mastering it will enable one of the most important leverage techniques in social dance. Leaders, if your hand directly covers the shoulder blade and your partner is slightly leaning back, your hand is on what's considered to be your partner's "center point of balance." If at any time your hand goes above or below this point, you'll lose control over your partner's body, and your partner will no longer feel secure. Go on, try it. Lower your hand about four or five inches and have your partner slowly lean backward the same way. Is she secure or comfortable? It's also good to know where your hand shouldn't be and why, so make sure you both understand so you don't accidentally fall into bad habits later.

Connection Point Three

Connection point 3 is typically the most visible part of a frame and the easiest to notice when it's not correct. This connection point includes the lady's left arm or elbow area and the man's right arm and/or elbow. Connection point 3 is typically only accomplished once the partners have established connection point 2.

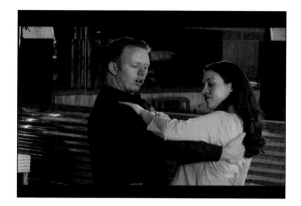

> **Connection point 1 is not needed for connection point 3 to take place. Connection point 3 does, however, almost always requires connection point 2.**

There should be a connection between the partners' arms or, in better terms, there should not be any space between the two partners' arms. Ladies, don't mistake this connection point for a well-placed arm rest; rather, you should treat it as yet another sensor to help you interpret your partner's bodily motions and plans. If the lady chooses to rest her arm completely on the man's, it is only a matter of seconds before the man removes his arm from the dance position because the weight typically becomes unbearable. Ladies, don't take it personally, but your arm—regardless of its size or weight—is heavy. Just know that anything additional on the leader's arm is heavy when the leader already has to support holding his own arm up and his shoulder is probably burning just to keep it in place.

Ladies, if the guy's right elbow is pointing downward to the ground rather than touching yours, do not leave yours up by itself. Drop your arm down just long enough to tap his elbow a time or two with yours, and then move it up. He should get the hint—if not, try it again. Try to avoid having great frame while your partner doesn't. Nothing is easier to spot than a follower holding her own on the floor when the man's posture or frame leaves something to be desired. Frankly, it just makes both of you look sloppy because the intent of social dancing is to look good as a couple, regardless of who you're dancing with.

Now try to put all three of the connection points together. First, start with connection point 1, then connection point 2, and then number 3. Now try just connection points 2 and 3. Excellent! Now, try the exercise where you close your eyes and go through the motions, but this time, use all three connection points. Does it feel different? It should be more secure. It'll get even better with the fourth one, coming up next.

Connection Point Four

Now it is time to complete your dance frame with connection point 4. Ladies, it is up to you to have correct placement with this final connection point. If you and your partner released from the previous three connection points, assemble your dance frame through connection point 3 at this time. Don't forget your soft knees and good posture.

Now that you are once again in connection points 1, 2, and 3, you're ready for the fourth. Ladies, place your left hand along your leader's right clavicle (collarbone). This should align the outside edge of your left hand, along the pinky, with the top edge of the leader's shoulder. The follower's wrist should fall somewhere in the area in front of the leader's right deltoid. Ladies have the option here to leave the entire hand in the front or, at a minimum, just the thumb; the reasoning will follow shortly.

> **Followers, if, after getting your left hand properly placed, your left elbow no longer aligns directly over your leader's elbow, don't panic. Proper placement of the hand supersedes direct elbow alignment in the chain of importance. If your elbow extends beyond your partner's, ladies, simply make sure there is connection between your arm and his arm in the areas where your arms align. Conversely, if your elbow does not reach your leader's elbow, simply create connection where your arms *do* meet. However, always hold your own weight. The leader is NOT an armrest!**

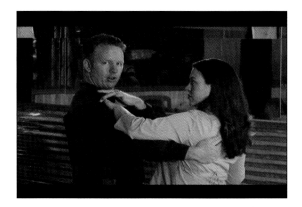

This connection point serves several purposes, including acting as a sensor for when the leader moves forward or back, and it allows the follower to maintain her personal dance space. First, having the hand or thumb in the front allows the follower to feel and react to either forward or backward motion. This is critical in leading and following because it allows for body positioning to help guide the partners, and is lost if the follower's hand is completely behind the shoulder blade. Second, if a leader is getting fresh or suffers from halitosis (bad breath), followers have the ability to hold the offending party at a more comfortable distance. Making the connection between the follower's left hand and the leader's right shoulder along the inside of the leader's body, rather than on top of or behind his shoulder, also physically forces your body into correct posture if you are applying the appropriate amount of tension to retain your dance space. As you push against the leader, you should feel your own shoulders being forced back and down, directly into the leader's hold at connection point 2.

Followers, proper alignment in connection point 4 should open your sternum toward the leader's face, allowing you to look him in the eye without dramatically tipping your head back or down, depending on your relative heights. This is advantageous in situations when you might be photographed or you might have an audience. Having the neck bent far forward or backward breaks the visual line from the tip of the toe to the top of the head and is much less visually appealing than when you are properly aligned.

A Fun Way to Practice the Connection Points

Now that you have felt a proper dance frame, use the following exercise to practice moving and maneuvering around a dance floor as a couple while in frame. To complete this exercise, you will need one hula hoop per couple dancing.

> **Needed: One hula hoop, two people, and a whole lotta fun!**

In this exercise you will be using the hula hoop to simulate a dance frame created with the four connection points. This exercise allows the leader to experience the sensations of the leads necessary to navigate the couple around the dance floor while locked into the proper frame. By using the hula hoop to create and support the dance frame between you and your partner, you are eliminating variables that complicate and occasionally impede your learning progress.

Following are the steps necessary to create your hula hoop dance frame.

1. Ladies, stand facing your partner.

2. Men, holding the hula hoop from the outside, place it over your partner's head so that it encircles her right below the armpits. It needs to catch her across the shoulder blades.

3. Ladies, take your arms around the outside of the hula hoop and wrap your hands around the hula hoop such that your elbows are either above or outside of the hoop, your forearms cross back underneath the hula hoop to the inside, your wrists are inside the hoop, and your fingers are holding onto the top side of the hula hoop. This locks the hula hoop in the proper position.

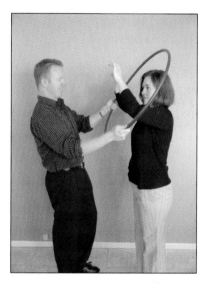

4. Men, make sure that you are holding the hula hoop from underneath, with your palms below the hoop and facing the ceiling and with your hands about shoulder-width apart.

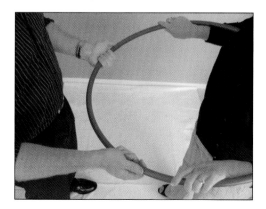

5. Keeping the two rules of the road in mind, men, put your weight on your right foot and prepare to step off with your left, and ladies, weight on your left foot, ready to step with the right.

6. Men, leading from your body, simply using your arms as extensions of your body, start moving around the floor. In other words, take your first step with your left foot, and as you do, if you are holding everything steady through your torso and arms, your follower should step automatically in the proper direction with her right foot.

7. Once you've mastered basic movements a step or so in every direction, start steering around the room.

8. If this begins to seem mundane, followers, close your eyes. Trust your dance partner's lead. If you can follow your partner with your eyes closed, you can be confident that you are truly following and your partner is truly leading.

9. Switch roles and start again at step 1.

Once you have mastered this exercise, continue on to the five basic foot positions.

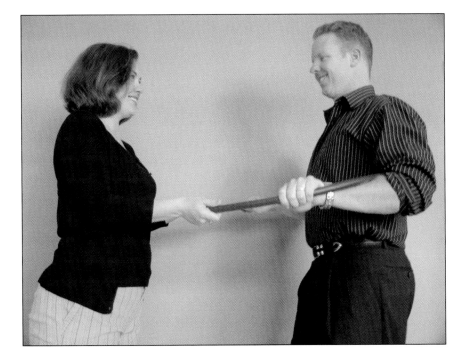

The Five Basic Foot Positions

T HERE ARE FIVE BASIC foot positions
that, if you learn them up front, will prove to
be extremely valuable to your learning progression. Sure, you can skip this section and go on
to something more fun, but understand that if you
spend a few minutes here figuring out what the
positions are, it will make going through each of
the step descriptions for the dances that much easier. It will provide a great visual reference point, or
cue, for you to go along with as you learn the
basics. In the following sections, each of the five
foot positions is broken down, as well as two
"extended" foot positions for you to go through.

First

First foot position is essentially having both of
your feet together, as the diagram shows. In many
dances, the first foot position is considered the
ready position because each partner will have weight
on one of the feet. (Ladies will have their
weight on the left foot, and men will have
their weight on their right foot, as discussed
in the two rules: Ladies are always right, and
men always get what's left.)

Remember: Feet together.

Second

Second foot position is the equivalent of having
your feet shoulder-width apart, or in a well-
balanced state. It is common to go into a second
foot position directly from a first foot position
when transitioning from one move to another
or just in executing side-steps, such as in slow
dancing or in the cha-cha, which you'll later learn.

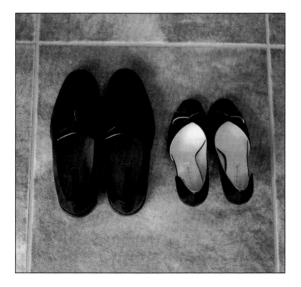

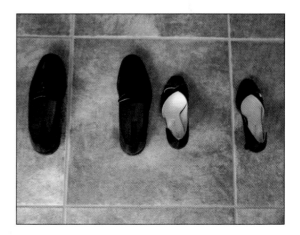

Remember: Feet shoulder-width apart.

Third and Extended Third

Third foot position is best described as "heel to instep." This is the equivalent of having one of your feet at a slight angle, pointed off of the center of your other foot. Third foot positions and extended third foot positions are used in almost every dance when creating the first step in a turn because they will allow one's body to create a new direction upon placing weight. Sometimes, the third foot position can also be used as a rock-step in swing, depending on the situation.

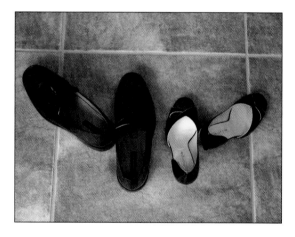

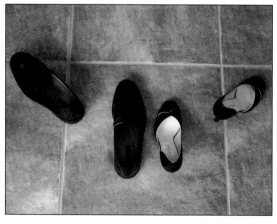

Remember: Heel to instep.

Fourth

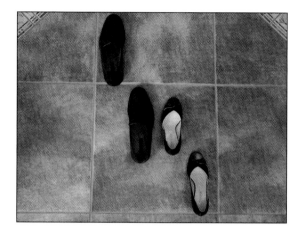

Fourth foot position is what you would do when walking down the street. It's what you should naturally go into when passing either foot in front of or behind the other in a straight line (straight forward or straight back). Fourth foot positions are often used in progressive dances, such as two-step and waltz (not the stationary waltz), but can also be used in dances such as the slow dance when simply moving forward and back with one's partner.

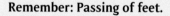

Remember: Passing of feet.

Fifth and Extended Fifth

Fifth foot position is what you are in when you have your toe just behind your heel. (It doesn't matter which foot is which.) It's best described as "heel to toe." Fifth foot positions and extended fifth foot positions are mostly used in swing dancing as the rock-steps because they allow the person to slightly open his or her hips and shoulders to a more dynamic position than just head-on with a partner.

Remember: Heel to toe.

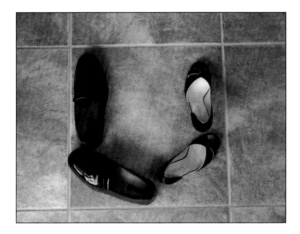 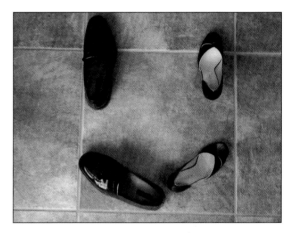

The five foot positions are the building blocks for almost every dance step you will ever learn. Clarity and confidence with these basic elements will accelerate your learning down the road.

The Six Dance Positions

N OW THAT YOU HAVE mastered the four connection points and the five basic foot positions, you have the necessities for constructing the six main dance positions. These dance positions are the building blocks for the various leads and moves you will learn in the dances taught in this text. As with other concepts taught in this chapter, an exercise is offered to cement these moves in your long-term memory prior to you moving on to the next step. As you master each of these pieces of dancing separately, the overall dance will fit together with ease, and you will be dancing proficiently much sooner than if you simply jumped in and tried to learn moves, footwork, lead and follow, rhythm, and styling all at once.

Open Dance Position

The open dance position is the most basic dance position and is, by definition, the simplest to create. However, despite the simplicity, this is a highly useful tool in your lead-and-follow toolbox. Several intermediate and advanced moves are based on the lead created by the open dance position.

Connection Points Used

There is no physical connection between the dance partners in the open dance position.

Foot Positions Used

All foot positions are used in the open dance position, which is usually started in first or second foot position.

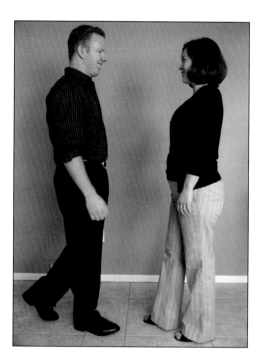

How to Create and Use the Open Dance Position

Stand facing your partner about one step (eighteen inches to two feet) apart without touching. Your shoulders should be parallel, and you should be facing each other squarely. You will be depending on a visual lead to execute coordinated movement between the lead and follow. This means that the follower must be watching the leader so each movement of the leader can be properly matched and balanced. This position is also called a *shine position* when the couple is executing a mirrored action. This is the easiest form of the dance positions to master. You will see the open (shine) position used in intermediate and advanced syncopations of several of the dances.

Syncopation is a deviation from the standard pattern. You can have syncopations in the rhythm of a step or in the way a step is executed. Syncopations are very popular in choreographed dances created for performance and competition.

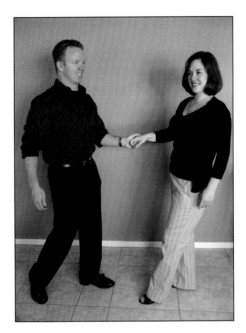

The open dance position is called the *challenge position* in the Latin dances, such as the cha-cha and salsa, when the dance partners release the physical connection points and dance back and forth in a call-and-response style. For example, the leader will release the lead and do a left turn by himself, while the follower holds the basic. Then, as the leader finishes his turn, the follower begins a corresponding left turn. This sequence continues until the leader changes from the open dance position to one of the five other dance positions and progresses to the next move.

One-Hand Hold

As we progress from the open dance position, the next logical step is the one-hand hold. Read on, and you will learn about this powerful and versatile connector.

Connection Points Used

The one-hand hold uses connection point 1.

Foot Positions Used

The one-hand hold uses all foot positions, and is usually started in first or second foot position.

How to Create and Use the One-Hand Hold

The one-hand hold describes a dance position in which one of the leader's hands is holding one of the follower's hands, either right or left. For example, the leader's left hand might be holding the follower's right hand, or the leader's right hand might be holding the follower's right hand. The one-hand hold is usually used for leading the follower into moves with lateral motion or rotational moves. The one-hand hold uses connection point 1, palm to palm. You will use the one-hand hold frequently in swing, West coast swing, salsa, and cha-cha.

The one-hand hold can be done with either hand of both the leader and the follower. The type of hand-hold varies from dance to dance and from move to move; it is not always palm to palm.

The four types of hand-holds used in this text are as follows:

- ▶ **The leader's left palm meets the follower's right palm perpendicular to the floor, at shoulder height.**

- ▶ **Either of the leader's palms is facing upward, held at about waist level, and the follower's opposite hand is placed in his.**

- ▶ **A handshake hold is created when a leader's right hand holds a follower's right hand, so a diagonal line is created between the two partners at waist level.**

- ▶ **In Latin dances, the one-hand hold is created by the leader holding his hand at chest level, elbow bent and fingers and thumb extended. The follower then wraps her opposite hand around the leader's thumb, and the leader gently closes his fingers over her hand. This hold is occasionally referred to as *Pac-Man* or *lobster claws*.**

Two-Hand Hold

The two-hand hold is the connection foundation for several moves in swing and Latin. This type of connection is also indispensable during the learning process as you and your partner match up your footwork.

Connection Points Used

The two-hand hold uses connection point 1.

Foot Positions Used

The two-hand hold uses all foot positions, and is usually started in first or second foot position.

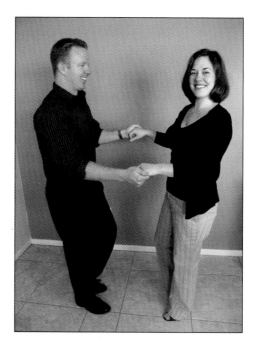

How to Create and Use the Two-Hand Hold

The two-hand hold is a combination of two one-hand holds. It is created by the leader standing facing his partner, with about 18 inches between them. In non-Latin dances, he raises his arms to waist level with his hands open (palms up) for the follower to place her hands into. The follower then places her hands in the leader's hands, and the leader gently grasps the follower's hands, being careful not to squeeze. In Latin dances, the leader holds his arms as described in the one-hand hold and uses a lobster-claw grip on both sides rather than just one.

It is imperative that the leader is careful not to squeeze in either the one-hand or two-hand holds. Ladies' hands can be bruised in these positions from overly zealous hand grips.

Closed Dance Position

The closed dance position is the quintessential dance position. It is usually the dance position that people associate with all couples dances.

Connection Points Used

The closed dance position uses connection points 1, 2, 3, and 4.

Foot Positions Used

The closed dance position uses primarily the first and second foot positions, but the fourth position is also used when the dance is progressive. The other foot positions are used as part of the steps.

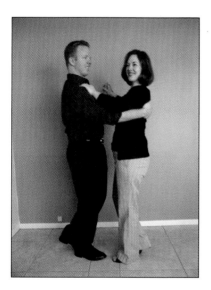

How to Create and Use the Closed Dance Position

You already created closed dance positions when you built your dance frame using all four connection points, so this should be fairly familiar to you. You will see and use the closed dance positions in each of the dances that are taught in this book and on the DVD. As a quick reminder, the closed dance position is built by the leader's left hand and follower's right hand connecting palm to palm, the leader's right hand connecting with the follower's left shoulder blade, the follower's left arm touching the leader's right arm in the elbow region, and the follower's hand (at minimum her thumb) held on the inside edge of the leader's shoulder, pressing up and away from him.

Promenade Dance Position

Promenade dance position is very similar to closed dance position. If you have seen tango danced, you have seen the promenade dance position.

Connection Points Used

The promenade dance position uses connection points 1, 2, 3, and 4.

Foot Positions Used

The promenade dance position uses primarily the third and extended third foot positions. The other foot positions are used as part of the steps.

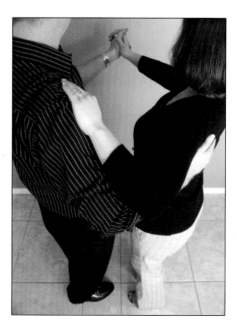

How to Create and Use
the Promenade Dance Position

Promenade position is also referred to as a *semi-open position*. It is a modified closed position because all four connection points are maintained; however, the leader and follower "open" their stance so they are no longer directly facing each other. Rather, they are both facing their connection at connection point 1. This creates a V shape with their shoulders, with the bottom point of the V at the leader's right and the follower's left elbow and the outside points of the V at the leader's left shoulder and the follower's right.

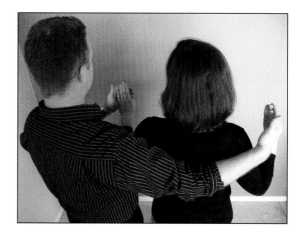

To create a promenade position, start in closed dance position. Change your feet so they are both in third position rather than first or second, with the leader's left toe pointed out to the left and the left heel near his right instep, and the follower's right toe pointed out to the right. This should naturally allow the leader's left hip and the follower's right hip to open to a 45-degree angle. Next, allow your shoulders to follow your hips. In swing, you would usually drop connection point 1 from shoulder level to waist level, with the leader's palm facing up and the follower's hand resting in the leader's. You are now ready to walk or dance forward together in the direction that the leader's left and the follower's right hands are pointing.

Sweetheart Dance Position

The sweetheart dance position is usually a means to an end. We doubt that you will ever execute an entire dance in sweetheart dance position, but if you advance in your dancing, particularly in two-step and swing, you will definitely utilize the sweetheart position.

Connection Points Used

The sweetheart dance position uses a variation of connection point 1.

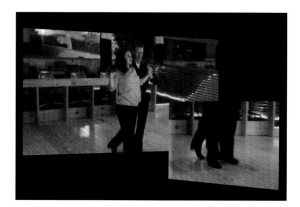

Foot Positions Used

The sweetheart dance position uses all foot positions.

How to Create and Use
the Sweetheart Dance Position

The sweetheart dance position is a side-by-side position in which the leader is typically on the left side and the follower is on the right, with both parties facing the same direction. To build the sweetheart position, both the leader and the follower must stand facing the same direction in first foot position. The follower should be slightly in front of the leader and off to his right. Her left shoulder should be in front of his right shoulder.

Followers, hold both of your hands up at shoulder level with the palms facing forward (in a "stick 'em up" position). You will be creating tension through pressing forward and out with both of your hands, so no spaghetti or collapsing arms are permitted in this position. Leaders, you will now take each of her hands in yours, right hand to right hand and left hand to left hand. Your fingers, held flat (not clenched), are pulling in toward you against her palms, and your thumbs are resting *gently* against the backs of her hands. This is so they aren't sticking up in an unsightly fashion.

As mentioned before, you are creating your dance frame through the connection in your hands—gentlemen, you should be pulling her in toward you, and you should feel her gently resisting. This tension will allow you to steer the two of you on the dance floor and allow her to sense your leads as you are not facing each other in this dance position. You will use this position frequently in the two-step, waltz, and other progressive dances. It is also nice to incorporate into slow dances when there are photographs involved.

Stop and Practice the Dance Positions

Now that you have incorporated foot positions with connection points to construct the six dance positions, it is time to create some muscle memory before you start adding fancy footwork to the dance positions.

The following exercise is designed to allow your bodies to adjust to these new positions. Take as much or as little time on it as you feel necessary—just remember, as simple as these positions seem now, if they are not fully concrete in your muscle memory, the minute you start adding footwork your frame will collapse and an adequate lead will become entirely out of the question. So, find a space that is big enough for you and your dance partner to walk 20 steps or so. This can be in a circle, around a room, or down a hallway. There also needs to be enough room for both of you to fit walking shoulder to shoulder. Next, at your starting point, assume the open dance position. Walk the length of the room or around the room, maintaining the open dance position. Try some lateral movement in each position as well. Some will be easier than others, but it'll be fun to go through them all. Repeat this exercise for each of the dance positions until you and your partner are completely comfortable.

Not every dance uses each of the six basic dance positions; however, mastery of all six dance positions will allow you to quickly and easily transition from basic to advanced patterns within the various dances.

Not all dancers are the same size and height. As you learn the basic dance positions, you will begin to see any adjustments that you will need to make to dance with your partner. For instance, if there is a large height differential, the closed dance position might not look exactly the same as it would with two people who are roughly the same height.

The Seven Essential Steps

THE FOOTWORK for every couples dance is composed of varying combinations of several dance steps. These dance steps are found in ballroom dance, country line dance, and other forms of individual dance, such as jazz, tap, and even ballet. The total list of dance steps is not infinite, and the number of steps used in the dances taught in this text is limited to seven. Read on to learn these by name and familiarize your feet with them. If you take the time to go through the following exercises and read the descriptions at this point in your dance education, you will expedite your learning curve as you progress with the dances. This section is designed to teach your feet what they need to be doing so your mind can stay busy with the more active pursuit of leading the dance with your partner. Each step includes a description as well as a brief exercise. It is strongly recommended that you and your dance partner practice each of these exercises as you go through. Some steps are more difficult than others, and mastery of the footwork is the key to success because it will allow you to focus on the lead-and-follow portion to complete each dance.

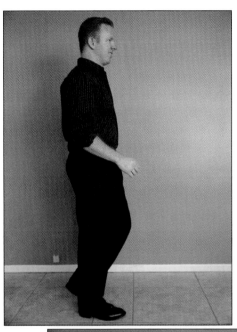

Walking-Steps

Walking-steps are exactly what they sound like. You use them to move forward and back without stepping to the right or left or crossing your feet. Picture yourself strolling down an unobstructed sidewalk with no obstacles in view; you can walk straight down this sidewalk with smooth, even steps, without stepping to the right or left.

Foot Positions Used

Walking-steps use the first and fourth foot positions.

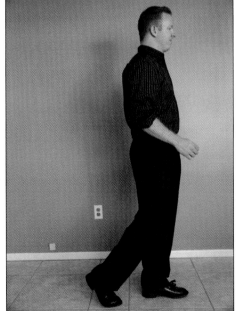

How to Do a Walking-Step

To take a walking-step with your right foot, begin in first foot position with your weight on your left foot. Step forward with your right foot to fourth foot position. Let your left foot pass your right to bring your feet to another fourth foot position, this time with your left foot ahead of your right. If you want to take walking-steps backward, you would begin with your weight on either your right or left foot, step behind you with the other foot to fourth foot position, and then let the first foot step back behind the second to another fourth foot position.

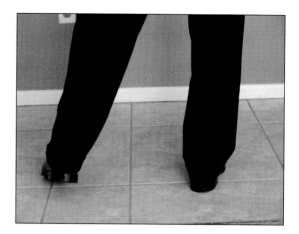

Master It Now

Take this opportunity to master walking-steps in both directions. Picture yourself back on the sidewalk mentioned before. Practice your walking-steps by taking eight steps forward, starting with either your right or left foot (depending on whether you're the leader or the follower), and then eight steps back. Repeat. Next, take four walking-steps forward, then four backward. Repeat. Cut down the number of walking-steps in each direction to two, and then one, and repeat. To get balanced practice, repeat the entire exercise by starting on the opposite foot than the one you started on.

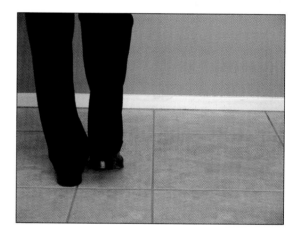

Side-Steps

Side-steps are exactly what they sound like. You use them to move to the right or left without stepping forward or backward or crossing your feet. Picture yourself in a movie theater—to slide down the row to your seat in the middle of the theater, you need to do side-steps.

Foot Positions Used

Side-steps use the first and second foot positions.

How to Do a Side-Step

A side-step to the right begins in first foot position with your weight on your left foot. Step out to the right with your right foot to second foot position. Let your left foot follow your right to bring your feet back to a first foot position, ready to begin your next side-step. If you want to side-step to the left, you would begin with your weight on your right foot, step to second foot position with your left foot, bring your right foot to meet your left in first position, and so on.

Master It Now

Take this opportunity to master side-steps in both directions. Picture yourself back in that movie theater. If there is a line on the floor that you can follow, it'll make it that much easier. Practice your side-steps by taking eight side-steps to the right, and then eight back to the left. Repeat. Next take four side-steps to the right and back to the left. Repeat. Cut down the number of side-steps in each direction to two, and then even one, and then repeat. You should do this exercise with both feet until you're comfortable.

Step-Touches

The name "step-touch" describes the two components of this particular step. You use them in stationary dances to create lateral movement and visual interest. Take the feeling of the single side-step back and forth and smooth out the motion. This is almost the step-touch.

Foot Positions Used

Step-touches use first and second foot positions.

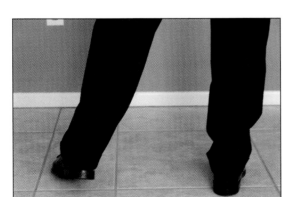

How to Do a Step-Touch

To step-touch to the right, begin in first foot position with your weight on your left foot. Step out to the right with your right foot, to second foot position. Let your left foot follow your right to bring your feet back to a first foot position. However, do not transfer your weight from the right to the left foot; instead, merely touch the left foot to the floor next to your right and prepare to step immediately back to the left. When you step-touch to the left, you begin with your weight on your right foot, step to second foot position with your left foot, bring your right foot to meet your left in first position without putting your weight down on the right foot, and prepare to step back to the left.

Master It Now

Take this opportunity to master step-touches. Do eight step-touches (a total of four to the right and four to the left) starting on each foot. As you practice, work on making these steps as smooth as possible.

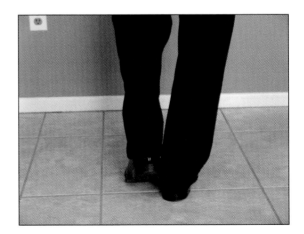

Tap-Steps

Have no fear; you will not be drilling metal plates onto the soles of your shoes and creating your own tap-dance routines. The tap-step simply refers to the weight change pattern in the step. A tap-step is also referred to as a *stutter-step*.

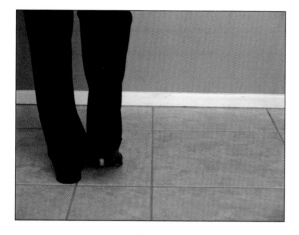

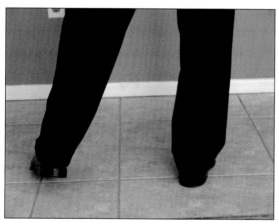

Foot Positions Used

Tap-steps use first and second foot positions.

How to Do a Tap-Step

A tap-step to the right begins in first foot position with your weight on your left foot. Step with your right foot as though you were going to take a step in place; however, do not change weight to the right foot, just tap it on the surface. Then, step again with the right foot, this time out to the second foot position, and transfer weight. To change directions and tap-step back to the left, once your weight is on your right foot, tap your left foot next to your right, and then step out to the left to the second foot position. If you want to do a tap-step to the left, you begin with your weight on your right foot and tap your left foot in first foot position, and then step with your left foot to second foot position.

Master It Now

Take this opportunity to master tap-steps. Do eight tap-steps (a total of four to the right and four to the left) starting on each foot. Do the tap-steps a few different times just to ensure you understand and can demonstrate the tapping first, then the change of weight.

Triple-Steps

Triple-steps are three quick steps taken in place, forward, backward, or to the side over two beats of music. So, if you were replacing two walks forward starting with your right foot with a right-forward triple-step, you would end up with an accelerated right-left-right in the same amount of time it would have taken you to do the original right-left. You will see these steps in a variety of dances; they are called *triple-steps* or occasionally *cha-cha-cha steps* in the Latin dances.

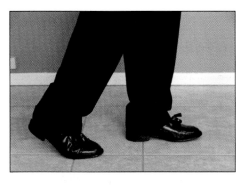

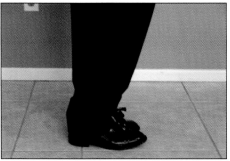

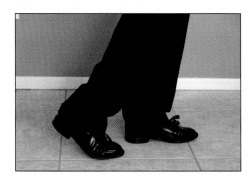

Foot Positions Used

Triple-steps use first foot position and second or fourth foot position.

How to Do a Triple-Step

As previously mentioned, a right triple-step forward is an accelerated right-left-right in the same amount of time two regular steps would have taken (two beats of music). A triple-step to either side rather than a regular side-step would be a side-together-side in the same amount of time it would take to do a side-together in a regular side-step. You can count this as tri-ple-step, one-and-two, right-left-right, pol-ka-step, shuf-fle-step, cha-cha-cha, and so on. The key is finding a naming method that makes sense to you.

Master It Now

Take this opportunity to master triple-steps in all four directions with either foot. Each time you complete a triple-step, try a different counting mechanism to find the one that works best for you.

Rock-Steps

Rock-steps are used to change direction or as a type of balance step when you are in a dance with a lot of lateral movement. Most of the dances that you learn in this text will incorporate a rock-step. The keys to successful rock-steps are control and restraint as you shift your weight.

Foot Positions Used

Rock-steps use first foot position and third, fourth, or fifth foot position.

How to Do a Rock-Step

You can rock-step forward or backward with either foot. To do a rock-step back with your right foot, begin in first foot position with your weight on your left foot. Bend your right knee and step back with your right foot to a fourth foot position. As your weight shifts briefly onto the ball of your right foot, straighten your right knee and bend your left knee. Then bend your right knee and step back forward onto your left foot. The particular dance that you are incorporating the rock-step into will dictate whether you shift your weight back to the right foot or keep your weight on the left foot with only a touch of your right foot. That being said, you will finish a rock-step in first foot position, regardless of which foot carries your weight.

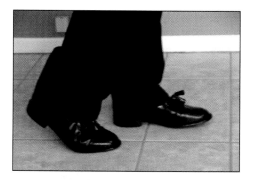

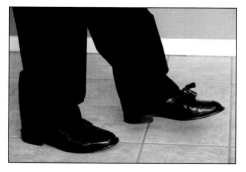

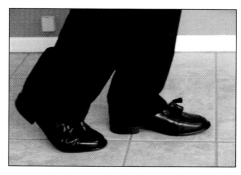

To rock forward you simply step forward into the fourth foot position with your right foot, and then back to first. To do a rock-step with your left foot, you begin with your weight on your right foot, flex your left knee and step back to fourth foot position with your left foot, then shift your weight back to the right foot, bending the left knee and bringing it back to first foot position with either a step or a touch (no weight change).

> **Please note that you will vary the type of foot position for your rock-step depending on the type of movement you are doing. If you are to remain squarely facing your dance partner for the move, you will rock back in fourth foot position, but if there is any opening of your frame to a promenade type of position, you will use a third or fifth position for your rock-step rather than the fourth. This allows you to open your shoulders and maintain alignment through your shoulders, hips, knees, and feet.**

Master It Now

Take this opportunity to master both forward and backward rock-steps with both your right and left feet. Starting with your weight on your left foot, rock back with your right, and then finish by putting your weight back on your left foot. When you complete your first rock-step, change your weight to the right foot and do a rock-step with your left. Make sure you avoid the two pitfalls of rock-steps—do not put your weight on your heel as you rock back, which causes you to lose control of your step, and do not leave your weight on your front foot and only touch your foot behind you. There must be a weight change; it just has to be a controlled one.

Anchor-Steps

Anchor-steps are specialized triple-steps that are used to ground a follower and create the necessary elastic tension in the West coast swing. If you have mastered the triple-step, you already have the timing for this step under your belt; it is just a matter of tackling the form of the step.

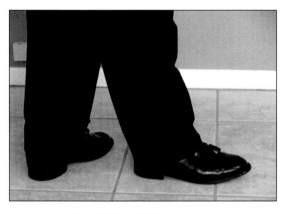

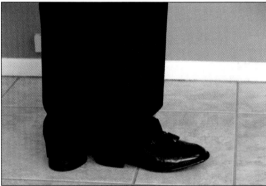

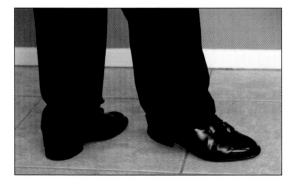

Foot Positions Used

Anchor-steps use first, third, and extended third foot positions.

How to Do an Anchor-Step

Although an anchor-step can be done with either foot, it will most frequently be done by the followers with the left foot and by the leaders with the right foot. Starting in first position with your weight on your right foot, step back into an extended third foot position with your left foot. This should have your left foot several inches (six or so) behind your right foot, with your right heel directly in line with your left instep and your left toes pointed out to the left at an angle between 45 and 90 degrees from your right foot. Step your right foot back into a third foot position, with your right foot pointing forward, left foot out to the side, and your right heel butting up against your left instep. You will finish the anchor-step by stepping back once again with your left foot into another extended third. This leaves you ready to start your next move with your weight on your left foot, ready to step with your right.

Anchor-steps are also sometimes taught with walking steps back in fourth position. Though it is also acceptable to do them in a fourth foot position, it is much more likely that you'll end up too far away from your partner, and the connection between the leader and the follower will be lost due to overextended arms. The use of the third and extended third foot positions opens your hips and shoulders to the side and allows you to create backward movement with your weight, a necessity for the strong West coast swing dance connection, while minimizing the total distance between you and your partner, preventing overextension of the arm connection.

Master It Now

You can practice anchor-steps best by yourself at first. Create a temporary dance partner by tying a T-shirt or towel to something stationary at about doorknob height. This will save wear and tear on your real dance partner and allow you to feel the tension connection that is a West coast swing trademark. Next, practice your anchor-steps holding on to the end of the towel that is not attached to your temporary dance partner. Concentrate on opening up your hips and shoulders as you move toward and away from your dance partner. Move away from your partner using anchor-steps, and move toward your dance partner with two walking-steps, right-left. The sequence should sound like either "right-left, an-chor-step" or "one-two, three-and-four" or "left-right, an-chor-step."

Understanding and knowing the name of each step will allow you to breeze through the individual footwork portions while you are learning the basics of each dance.

The Eight Directional Possibilities

THERE ARE EIGHT directional possibilities for movement on any dance floor. They include the following:

► **Forward**

► **Front-right**

► **Right**

► **Back-right**

► **Back**

► **Back-left**

► **Left**

► **Front-left**

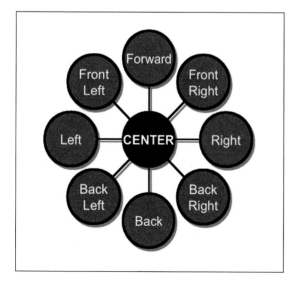

Practice the directional possibilities by marking out a square between 12 and 18 inches wide. If you have a tile floor, use the pattern to create your square. If you don't have a tile floor or other ready box pattern, you can create a box on your floor with some masking tape. Once you have your box, stand in it in first position. With your weight on your right foot, step forward to fourth foot position. Step back into your box to first. Next, step front-right into extended third. Step back. Step out to the right into second foot position. Return to first foot position. Step back-right, and then return to the first position. Step directly back into fourth foot position. Return to first. Continue with your weight on your left foot and step with your right foot to the back-left. This is a form of an extended fifth foot position, as your right toe should align with your left heel and your right heel should be pointing to the back left. Return to first position. Cross your right foot behind or in front of your left to step all the way to the left. Return to center with first foot position. Cross your right foot in front of your left to the front-left. Return to center. Now, shift your weight onto your right foot and, using your left foot, step in each of the directional possibilities going counterclockwise around your center box, remembering to return to first foot position between each step.

Leading and Following

"WHAT DO YOU EXPECT me to follow when there's no lead?" This is just one very common statement out on the dance floor. Another often-used one is, "If you're not going to lead me, I'm not going to move." Leading and following can be described as very advanced methods of communication because both sides need to understand their own roles and responsibilities as well as the other person's, and this has to be achieved using nonverbal communication, with only occasional exceptions. Without a doubt, the ability to lead or follow is skill-based, not just something people are born with. This should be good news to you if you're thinking right now that there is no way you'd ever be able to lead or follow someone. In just a moment, you'll read about and explore what both partners need to know about both leading and following. Don't just read the leading part if you're the leader or the following part if you're the follower. It's critical to understand both so you know how it all comes together.

Rules for Social Dancing

Followers	Leaders
Don't hang on.	Don't let her hang on.
Don't let go.	Don't let her let go.
Don't think.	Don't give her the chance to think.

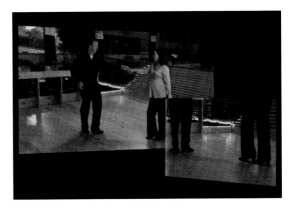

Following

Followers, if you have been skimming this chapter thus far, stop skimming. It is imperative that you master these rules before you advance in your dancing.

Don't Hang On

The follower's role is a role of sensitivity and finesse. Your main role is to grace the dance floor with your beauty and your dance partner with your presence. In this vein, clinging to your partner should be out of the question—it is neither attractive nor controlled. Your responsibility is one of availability—your hands should be available and ready for the leader's next signal. If you are in a closed dance position, release your vise-like grip on the leader's left hand and right shoulder. Be prepared to turn or release completely at his subtle prompt. If you are coming out of a turn or returning to a closed dance position or two-hand hold, do not under any circumstances reach and try to grab his hands. Make yours available at waist level so he can easily pick up your hand. If both of you are grasping for the other, chances are you will both miss on the first try. Let him do his job, while you focus on yours.

Don't Let Go

Though initially the first and second rules seem contradictory, they are not. Social dance is a balancing act, and following is no exception. Although you should not be clinging to your partner like a barnacle to a boat, you should not be so light and wispy that you float away altogether. The connection necessary for a lead is created by tension, and that tension in turn is created by contact between you and your leader. As a follower you need to stay connected to your leader at all costs by supporting your portion of the dance frame and providing resistance when appropriate.

Don't Think

This is the most challenging rule for followers. It is so difficult to master that many seasoned followers fail to relinquish their lead-hijacking ways on the dance floor. This rule does not mean that you should check your brain at the ballroom door or that following is a mindless activity. On the contrary, following requires a great deal of concentration and skill. As such, your mind should not be occupied with thinking about the next move coming up or predicting what the leader will do next. This consumes your thinking and doesn't allow you to respond to his real lead. Rather, your mind should be occupied with the rhythm of the dance, your basic footwork, and concentrating on listening with your whole body to your leader, sensing his nonverbal cues as he leads. As he is learning to lead, it is also your job to focus on the leads and give him feedback to improve them.

Leading

Leaders, this is your section. Read the following rules carefully and take them to heart. These rules apply to each and every social dance that you will learn.

Don't Let Her Hang On

The leader's role is self-defining. The leader is in charge on the dance floor, and subsequently responsible for holding and supporting his dance partner within the dance frame. Whether your follower has spaghetti arms or responds to your ease with the sensitivity of a cement truck, you are the one to hold her. She should not feel as though she needs to hold onto you; rather, she should be providing tension against you. When you are transitioning between moves and going in and out of turns or reconnecting after releasing a hand-hold, you are the one to reach for her hands. You are responsible for knowing where to look for those hands and being assertive with your lead.

Don't Let Her Let Go

Hand in hand with your responsibility to prevent her from hanging on is your responsibility to prevent her from letting go. As the leader, you have been designated as the initiator of each move. It is your job to release your partner at the proper time in a move; don't allow her to simply slip out of your dance frame. Along the same vein, when you are holding her, hold securely, but a vise grip is not acceptable. If you have an iron grip, the dance floor is not the place to show it. You will leave bruises, which leads to unpopularity on the dance floor among followers.

Don't Give Her the Chance to Think

This last responsibility of the leader is the most challenging for beginning dancers. It is what makes a good leader an incredible dance partner.

A proficient leader is always thinking about two moves ahead with a constant eye for changes in the composition on the dance floor that could impact his plans. It is the leader's job to think and execute so the follower doesn't have the chance or opportunity to think. If you stay in one move too long, chances are your partner will get bored and start stealing your hard-earned lead. Or, worse, she will stop paying attention to your lead and miss your next signal.

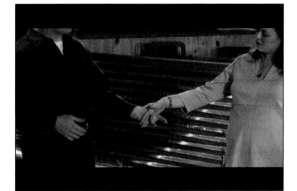

These rules of leading and following are based on the lines of communication between two dancers on the dance floor. It is imperative that each of you understands both your role and your partner's role to succeed as a couple on the social dance floor.

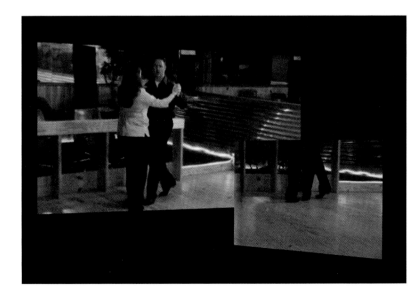

Putting It All Together

THIS CHAPTER has been spent filling your dance toolbox with the nuts and bolts of social dance. You have been exposed to the two basic rules for starting a social dance, the three R's of surviving partner dancing, the four connection points, the five foot positions, the six dance positions, the seven essential dance steps, and the eight directional possibilities. Combined with the short course on dance etiquette and the nitty-gritty of leading and following, this made for a packed learning experience. Take this opportunity for a quick recap before diving into the slow dance. Tattoo these foundation concepts to your memory before progressing to the individual dances.

▶ Remember the rules of partner etiquette—don't give unsolicited advice, thank your partner, and always introduce yourself.

▶ The rules of floor etiquette include being aware of your surroundings, apologizing or excusing yourself, and knowing the proper placement on the dance floor.

▶ The two rules for starting any ballroom dance are ladies are always right, and men always get what is left.

▶ The three R's of social dance are Respect for self, Respect for others, and Responsibility for all actions.

▶ The four connection points are palm to palm, palm to shoulder blade, elbow to elbow, and collarbone to palm.

Although not previously mentioned, if you are in a country-western nightclub, it is also important to know that if the DJ has designated a song as a line-dance song, couples dancing is only welcome around the periphery of the dance floor if space allows. In the same vein, if a song has been designated as a couples dance—for instance, West coast swing—line dancers are only welcome on the floor if there is space, and then off to the side, allowing plenty of room for the social dance and dancers.

Leaders, if you do not feel your partner leaning back into your lead and you are connected at connection point 2, you can use the following nonverbal signal to remind her to lean back into your hand. If she is not leaning back into your hand in such a way that you can clearly feel her shoulder blade and lead her effectively with just your right hand, take the fingers of your right hand without moving your palm and lightly tap your fingers along her back to silently and discreetly request that she lean back into your hand.

▶ The five foot positions are feet together, feet shoulder-width apart, heel to instep, a walking-step, and heel to toe.

▶ The six dance positions are open, one-hand hold, two-hand hold, closed, promenade, and sweetheart. These are created with various combinations of connection points and foot positions.

▶ The seven essential dance steps are walking-steps, side-steps, step-touches, tap-steps, triple-steps, rock-steps, and anchor-steps.

▶ The eight directional possibilities are forward, forward-right, right, back-right, back, back-left, left, and forward-left.

▶ The basic rules of leading are don't let the follower hang on, don't let her let go, and don't give her the chance to think.

▶ The basic rules of following are don't hang on, don't let go, and don't think.

You are now fully equipped and ready to start learning to dance. Keep in mind that everything you will learn in this text is based on different combinations of the steps, dance positions, connection points, and directional possibilities that you learned in this chapter. Also, the rules of etiquette and leading and following bear remembering because they will sustain you through the remainder of this text and the full course of your social-dancing career.

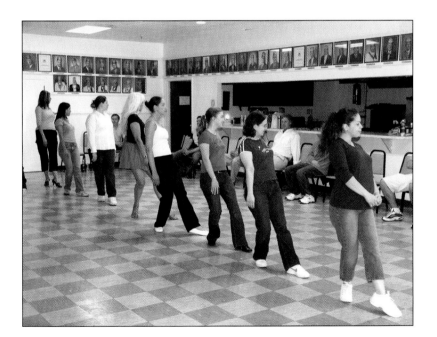

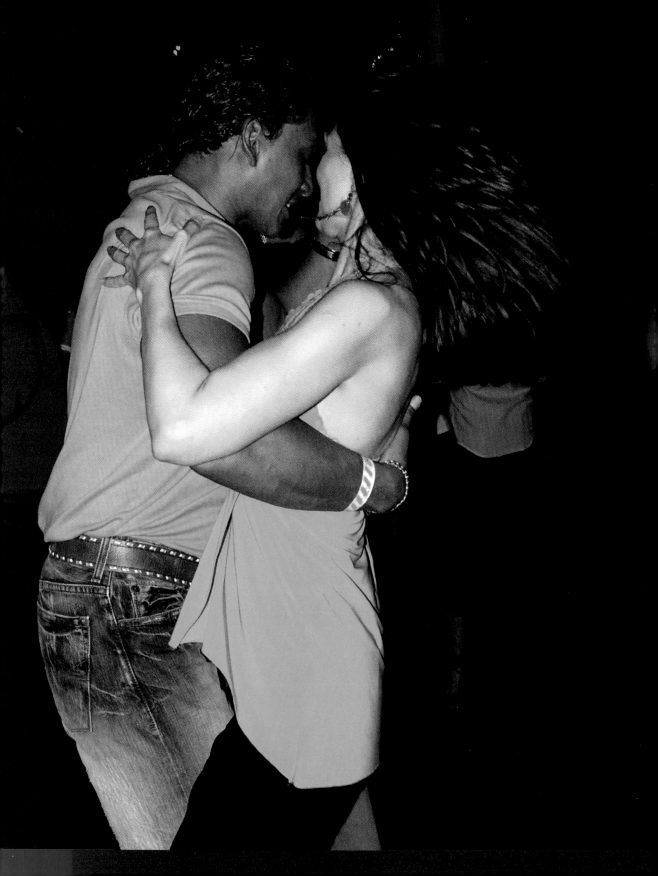

3

Picture Yourself
Slow Dancing

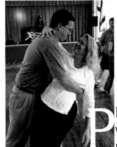

PICTURE YOURSELF and your dance partner walking out to the center of the dance floor. It might be your 30th anniversary, a romantic evening, or a quiet moment at home with good music. On the more formal end of the spectrum, it might be your wedding day, and now that the vows have been exchanged and the rings are on the fingers, it is time to celebrate with that memorable first dance. Your new bride is on your arm, smiling, looking more beautiful than you have ever seen her. You are feeling very sharp yourself in your tuxedo—who knew you were that tall when you stood up straight? As you reach the center of the floor, the moment arrives. You gently take your wife's hand from your arm, lift it, and spin her out away from you, only to draw her back in and begin your dance. You confidently lead her through your first dance, moving around the floor, spinning her, and finishing the moment with a picture-perfect dip, all captured by your videographer and photographer. Your wife is beaming as you two return to your table and continue the festivities as the cheers from your friends and family members slowly subside.

The Six Ws of Slow Dance

A S YOU'LL RECALL from Chapter 1, there are six Ws of dance: who, what, where, when, why, and wear. The following sections will walk you through the six Ws of slow dance.

Who Popularized Slow Dance?

Slow dancing is a distinctly American tradition that has been adopted by some other cultures along with the music it accompanies. No particular individual can be credited with the popularization of contemporary slow dancing; rather, it was popularized by a generation and a type of music. The youth of every era redefine slow dancing for their contemporaries as they shape their musical tastes.

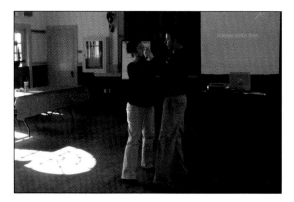

What Is Slow Dance?

Slow dancing is meant to be an impromptu romantic escape from the mundane for two people. In its most basic form, the slow dance you frequently see is the standard "cling and sway." Occasionally, an adventurous leader will heat it up by wobbling around in a circle while he and his partner cling to each other. This basic form is typified by the follower's arms draped around the leader's neck and the leader's arms either clasped conservatively around the follower's waist or, if he is feeling a bit fresh, they might reach down to her derriere. As intimate as this form of dancing is for the participants, it is downright boring to watch.

This is where the Slow Dance for Romance comes into play. The Slow Dance for Romance taught in this text and on the accompanying DVD, and in Shawn Trautman's *Learn to Dance* series, specifically on the *Couples Ultimate Dance Sampler*, takes "cling and sway" to a whole new level, making graceful and deliberate lead-and-follow dancing attainable for every beginner. This combination of leadable moves and simple footwork makes a mundane slow dance into a romantic event to remember both for the dancers and for anyone who has the pleasure of being an audience.

Where Did Slow Dance Originate and Where Is It Typically Done?

As mentioned previously, slow dancing is an American tradition that has subsequently spread to other cultures, accompanying the music to which it is danced. There is no specific geographic region within the United States that can be credited with the creation of the slow dance.

Slow dancing is done in myriad settings. The slow dance being taught in this chapter is appropriate in the nightclub setting; at a dance; at a formal event, such as a reunion or a wedding; or even in the privacy of your own living room. The slow dance taught in this text is as enjoyable to dance as it is to watch.

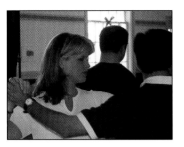

When Did Slow Dance Become Popular and When Is the Right Time to Slow Dance?

The slow dance as we know it today emerged in the 1960s, when dancing to popular upbeat music (versus slow and romantic ballads) shifted from couples dancing to solo dancing where men and women danced together, but touching was discouraged and individuality was encouraged. There was a shift in emphasis from rhythm to lyrics when appreciating contemporary Top 40 music. The '60s also marked the advent of rock concerts, where dancing became nothing more than swaying back and forth. This is the root of today's slow dance. The slow dance taught in this text takes the

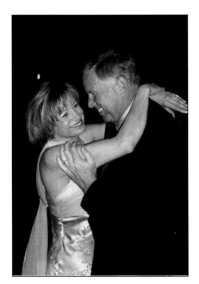

simplicity of the root slow dance just described, adds additional movement through simple footwork, and incorporates leads and moves from a variety of dances to add interest and zest to a simple and romantic slow dance.

Slow dancing is appropriate on innumerable occasions. Because of the simplicity of the dance taught in this text, it is extremely versatile and can be used in any genre of romantic music, be it soft rock, country, Latin, Top 40, or any one of many others. If you are a beginner social dancer, the appropriate time to learn to slow dance is now. You will be learning the basics of lead-and-follow dancing as well as moves that you will use in more intricate dances to the slower tempo and simple footwork of the slow dance.

Why Is the Slow Dance Danced?

The slow dance is danced as an intimate and romantic interlude between the two dancers. It is

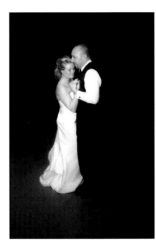

a dance of romance rather than passion or desire, like the rhumba or tango. It is more intimate than the waltz and is more appropriate on occasions when the waltz is too stylized or formal. It is also a romantic dance created to accompany the 4/4 timing of contemporary music.

©istockphoto.com/Justin Horrocks

What Kind of Attire Should Be Worn?

There is no dress code or standard apparel for the slow dance. Whatever you happen to be wearing when you are with your dance partner and the right song starts playing is perfectly appropriate.

Visualize the Slow Dance

SOMETIMES CONCEPTUALLY it's hard to get a good feel for what you're attempting to learn until after you see someone else doing it. Once you've seen it, you allow your mind to start processing ideas about how to get your body to do the same thing. Before we get into the nuts and bolts of how to slow dance, take a few minutes to turn on your DVD player and view the section entitled "Slow Dancing."

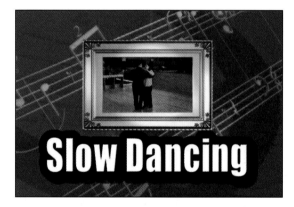

It's best if you watch the section one time through without trying to do any of it. Just give your mind a chance to absorb the material so it's somewhat familiar to you when you replay the section. Watch how the dancers move, think about the words that are used, and picture yourself doing the slow dance.

The second time you go through it, take notes. Begin to jot down the important parts of the dance so you can engage other parts of the kinesthetic learning prior to getting up and dancing along. Write down what the connection points are, what the basic steps are called, how many counts are in a basic, how to align with your partner, and so on.

Also, write down any questions that you might have at this point. There's a good chance you will find the answer later on in this chapter, and if it's something you're already pondering, you're sure to remember the answer for the long-term.

You'll find that by time you get ready to stand up and try the DVD, the dancing won't be nearly as overwhelming. Writing down the key concepts will allow you to get a jumpstart on the rest of the chapter. You'll also find that after you get up and try it, you'll probably have more questions. As this chapter goes on, the steps will be broken up with screenshots from the DVD, pointers will be given on where you should be during different parts of the dance, and frequently asked questions will be addressed that should satisfy most (if not all) of your questions, and then some.

The third time you view the DVD, go ahead and dance along with it. See how far you can make it just by watching and trying. You'll probably find that one of the two of you is able to pick up and understand the material quicker than the other.

> **Just remember, everyone learns at a different pace. Be cognizant of this as you're learning with your partner. One of you might pick up certain aspects of the dance quicker than the other, and that's okay. Try to be patient and wait for the other person to grasp the material, and then move on.**

Now, take a look at the rest of these pictures. All of them are taken of couples slow dancing. Some are formal and some are very informal, but the couples are all doing the same steps. See whether you can visualize yourself slow dancing (the dance you just watched over and over) in all these different settings. Then, picture yourself slow dancing at events you have coming up or at local venues where you and your partner can go. If you can see it, you can do it.

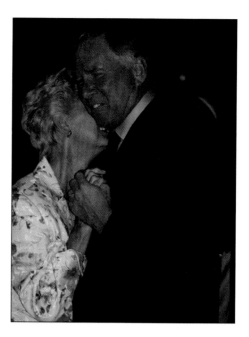

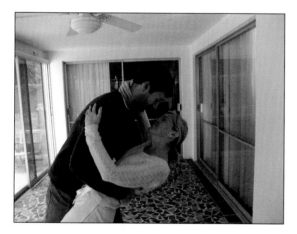

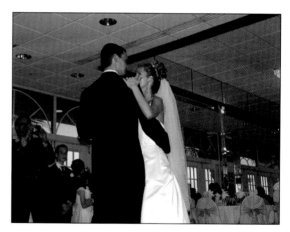

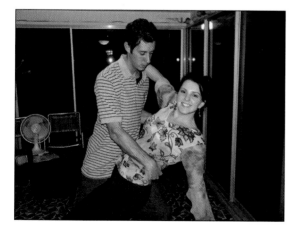

Slow Dance Basics

BEFORE WE GET too far down the road here, let's make one thing perfectly clear: *All* slow songs can include a nice, elegant, and romantic slow dance. (In other words, there's no song too slow to dance a slow dance to.) There might be songs that feel better to dance to and might even be easier to dance to, so let's just say that all songs qualify. For practice purposes for this dance, you can turn the radio on to whatever your favorite station is and "assume the position." Dance to anything and everything up front until you get familiar with the basics and feel good about the leading and following portions. Having said all that, let's get into the dance.

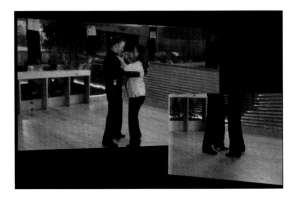

But first, let's not forget the two most important rules:

1. Ladies are always right! Ladies, put your weight on your left foot so you can be ready to start with your right. (This is what's called your *ready position*.)

2. Guys always get what's left. Guys, put your weight on your right foot so you can be ready to start with your left. (This is your *ready position*.)

The Four-Count Basic

The four-count basic of slow dancing is made up of two sets of steps and touches, or *step-touches*. In layman's terms, it's said out loud like this:

Step, touch, step, touch

If you're more mathematically inclined and like to use numbers, it's counted like this:

One, two, three, four

> **In the four-count slow dance basic, each step or touch consists of only one count— nothing more, nothing less. It's very even and smooth, which helps people who have very little rhythm.**

To try the slow-dance basics in place, assume foot position 1 and be in your ready position.

1. First step down with your free foot. Make sure you change weight on this one.

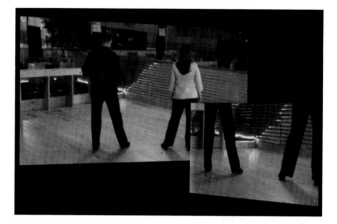

2. Using just the toe of the foot that is now free, touch down beside the other foot. Make sure you do not change weight to the toe you're touching with.

3. Lift that toe off the ground momentarily after Step 2, and then step back down onto it with a definite change of weight.

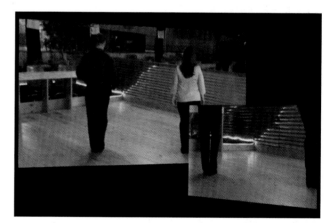

4. Just like in Step 2, use just the toe of the foot that is now free and touch down beside the other foot. Again, make sure you do not change weight to the toe you're touching with on this one.

Now that you're able to do these steps in place, let's go ahead and move a little bit with them.

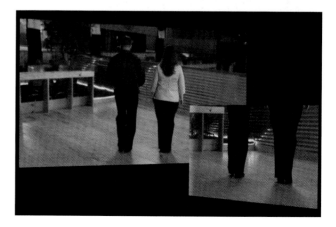

Try it moving back and forth over and over, doing step-touches. Steps 1 and 3 both use foot position two (FP2), and Steps 2 and 4 use foot position one (FP1). Leaders, your first step is to the left, about shoulder-width or so apart, and followers, your first step is to the right. Try not to be stiff-legged in this one as you start to move. Relax and enjoy.

Mirroring

Go ahead and face each other, giving yourselves anywhere from about two to five feet of space in between. You should now be in open dance position. The very first thing we'll go through will require the leader to move off to each of the eight directional possibilities, and the follower will attempt to mirror him. As you are probably envisioning right now, this means that as the leader takes a single step to his left while still facing the follower, the follower then takes the same-sized step to her right. The "identical" movement that the follower creates is called *mirroring*, and it's part of the "visual" aspect of following.

Leaders, go ahead and take a step with your left foot. This is not an exercise in trying to trick your partner by moving at the last second; rather, it is one where trust is starting to be built. Do the slow-dance basic footwork, and this exercise should not be a problem. Each time it is started, the leader should start with his left foot and the follower should start with her right.

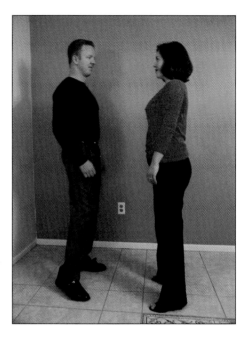

Leaders, feel free to test any one of the eight directional possibilities with your first step. Naturally, the second foot or step for the leader should be in the exact opposite direction to take him back to center. For example, if the leader steps forward on the first step, then he should step backward on the second; if the leader steps front-left on the first step, he should step back-right on the second.

> **If either partner gets on the "wrong foot" or goofs up during the exercise, just stop, laugh, and start back up again after the leader counts it off... 5-6-7-8, and you're back dancing again.**

Next, try to do this exercise to music. Almost any song will work, so go ahead and pick your favorite. It'll be the last thing you try before putting it all together and dancing for the first time. Leaders, you might want to count out loud to give the follower a chance to match you step for step when you start. This means the leader will say "5-6-7-8" and then step with his left foot. Another option is to say "Ready, and" or "Ready, set," which effectively takes the place of numbers 7 and 8. Leaders, try a few of these starting points and see which one you're comfortable with.

The Four-Count Basic as a Couple

Now that you're both experts on doing the basics on your own and in all the different directions, it's time to try them together. Hopefully you completed the exercise on the previous page and didn't just skip right to the dancing. If you skipped right to the dancing and didn't practice it on your own, you might have a tough time figuring out where any problems are if they arise. Practicing before coming together is critical to building the confidence of each partner and, especially if this is your first dance, you want to come in with high expectations. Social ballroom dancing is probably close to 25-percent skill and 75-percent attitude, so we hope you're in good spirits moving forward here.

Your toolkit for the slow-dance basics includes:

▶ **Foot position 1 (ready position and counts 2 and 4 of the basic)**

▶ **Foot position 2 (counts 1 and 3 of the basic)**

▶ **Connection points 1–4 (all will be used here in the basic)**

▶ **Four-count basic (essential for the slow dance to work)**

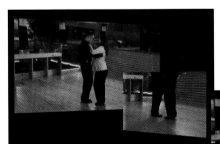

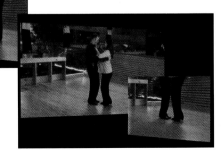

Okay, let's get into position and get this show started. The first thing you want to do is get into your dance position with your partner (use all four connection points) and be in your ready position. Leaders, go ahead and give your countdown (5-6-7-8) and move off to your left and then back to your right, and then repeat it over and over. Okay, you're doing the basics now. . .step, touch, step, touch, step, touch, step, touch. . . . Great job!

Now, let's juice it up a bit. This time when you go to try it, let's have the leaders actually lead it. By leading, we're not talking about verbal leads; we're talking about through the body. Leaders, when you're ready, let's see whether we can put this together and make it work. You have four connection points that you will use here to help you out. The two most important ones to start the dance will be connection points 1 and 2. Leaders, your left and right hands must be in sync on this one because both of them are necessary to provide guidance for the follower. A simultaneous movement of both of hands in equal force to your left at the same time that you step will get your partner moving. Give it a shot.

Did it work? If so, you did each of the following things. (You should aim for at least two of the three.)

▶ **You successfully transferred her weight from her left foot to her right.**

▶ **You managed to keep her directly in front of you.**

▶ **You kept a smile on her face or caused one.**

Did you realize that when you were leading her to the left, you used the palm of your right hand more than anything else? Remember, it has to be equal between the two hands. Truly, if the follower is able to feel your hands at all and she doesn't feel like she's nicely fastened and on some kind of a ride, it might need some work.

Regardless, now that she's here, you have to get back to the other side where you started. This time, leaders, instead of using your left hand and the palm of your right hand, you want to use your left hand and the fingers of your right hand. The left hand remains steady, yet it moves to the right and the fingers, together (not digging into her skin), will gently pull (guide) her back to the right if you're cupping her shoulder blade appropriately. Now, as she moves off to the right heading back toward the starting point, where her weight would change to her left foot, you, as the leader, want to slow her momentum down by using the palm of your right hand—sort of a nice cushiony landing, just to start back up again.

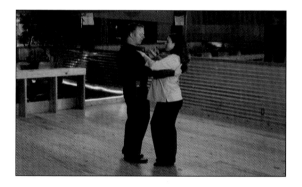

For the Followers

Followers, this next part might be difficult to comprehend because you probably want to help, but try your best. If the leader isn't perfectly clear on the lead (in other words, the motion or the guidance), don't move! You don't want to be stubborn and just stand there, but if the lead isn't nearly perfect, make him improve it. There shouldn't be much of an argument here—either you feel it and it's enough or you don't. The only major thing you need to focus on here is being in good frame and sitting slightly back into connection point 2.

For the Leaders

Leaders, listen up. If you give a lady a choice (on the dance floor), she'll take it! If you leave the door open for interpretation, you never know what you'll end up with. Nothing personal here, ladies; it would be the same if you were leading. Okay leaders, take your partner in your arms in closed dance position (with the four connection points, of course) and try the basics again. Try it over and over and practice the leads going both directions. Have your follower close her eyes and see whether she can follow what you're doing. If you're leading correctly, your partner will match your speed and do exactly what your body tells her to do. If the follower is having difficulty, there's a better than 90-percent chance it has something to do with the lead.

Followers, be sure to let the leader set the tempo on the dance floor. It is more important that the two of you dance together than to the beat of the music. If the leader is dancing to the beat of his own drum, or at least a beat not discernible to you, follow him anyway. The worst thing that will happen is a true critic might look at the two of you and wonder whether they are hearing the beat correctly. If you try to correct your partner in the middle of the dance, or worse, start dancing to a different beat, it will become painfully obvious that one of the two of you is off beat and that you aren't dancing together.

Remember that ladies are always right, and men always get what's left.

The Basics in All Directions

Now that you're both experts on doing the basics from side to side, you'll find that you might soon get bored, if you haven't already. What you'll do now is move not only from side to side, but also forward and back and at diagonals. (You'll use your eight directional possibilities on these.) The step-by-step guide is broken down for leaders and followers separately, but you should both try to learn the opposite footwork to give you a better perspective of what's happening with your partner.

For the Leaders: Part 1

Leaders, on your next basic you'll step front-left on the first count (extended third foot position), tap your right foot together on two (first foot position with your weight still on your left foot), and then step back-right with your right foot on three (back to the extended third foot position again), and then tap your left foot together on four (back to the first foot position), which brings you back into the ready position to start a new direction. Below is the visual depiction of your steps.

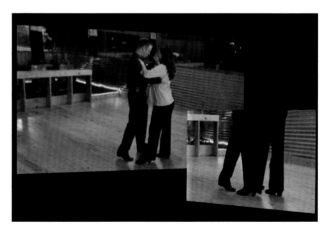

For the Followers: Part 1

Followers, your steps are the exact opposite on this one. You're going to step back-right on the first count, tap your left foot together on two (first foot position with your weight still on your right foot), and then step front-left with your left foot on three, and then tap your right foot together on four (back to the first foot position), which brings you back into the ready position to start a new direction. At the right is the visual depiction of your steps.

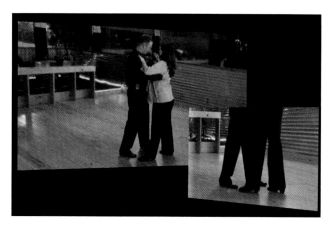

New Dimension to the Lead

When you were just going side to side in the four-count basic, the majority of the lead came through connection points 1 and 2, whereas connection points 3 and 4 were just along for the ride and to keep you looking good. With these next steps, all four connection points become engaged. Leaders, connection point 3 (your right elbow) will be slightly lifted (an inch or two) in order to shift your follower's weight from a balanced perspective to one where her weight is now in motion backward. This should cause her to take a backward step when she moves. In addition, the leader will be stepping toward the follower, triggering connection point 4 on the inside edge of the leader's right shoulder. Followers should feel pressure on their left hand and, in order to maintain their frame, they should then want to move backward to keep the proper distance. In contrast, by slightly dropping the elbow (connection point 3), the leader allows the follower's weight to shift toward the elbow, which makes it easier to lead steps in which you need the follower to move toward you (in other words, you're stepping back in some direction).

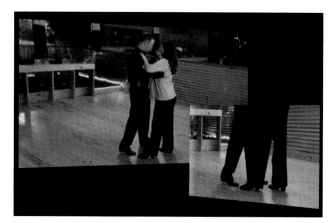

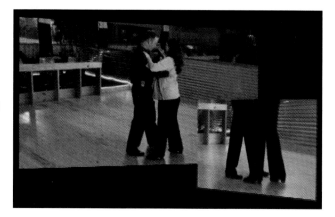

For the Leaders: Part 2

You'll now add onto what you just learned in Part 1. After you get back into a ready position from doing the four counts going front-left, you'll go back-left. The steps are broken down as follows.

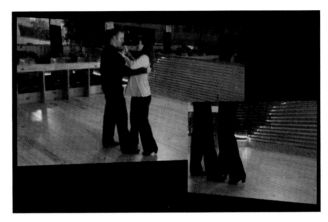

Leaders, on your next basic you'll step back-left on the first count, tap your right foot together on count two (first foot position with your weight still on your left foot), and then step front-right with your right foot on three (back to the extended third foot position again), and then tap your left foot together on four (back to the first foot position), which brings you back into the ready position to start a new direction. At the right is a visual depiction of the steps.

For the Followers: Part 2

Followers, your steps are the exact opposite on this one. You're going to step front-right on the first count, tap your left foot together on two (first foot position with your weight still on your right foot), and then step back-left with your left foot on three, and then tap your right foot together on four (back to the first foot position), which brings you back into the ready position to start a new direction. At the right is a visual depiction of the steps.

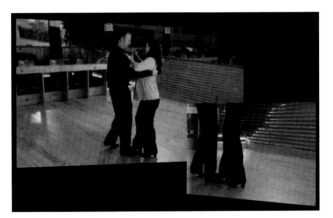

Mixing Up the Directions for Practice

Leaders, it's now up to you to start putting a few pieces together to test out your lead. Under your belt, you now have a number of steps that you can execute in almost any order as long as you start with your left foot, and only after completing a basic with your right foot.

The steps that you can mix up and try in any order include:

> ▶ **Side basics (left and right)**

> ▶ **Front-left basic**

> ▶ **Back-right basic**

> ▶ **Back-left basic**

> ▶ **Front-right basic**

The side basics (left and right) are what you should consider your default basic. If at any time during the dance the leader cannot think of anything else to do or just wants to take it easy for a moment, these are the steps that should be done. Then, at any point after completing a basic, the leader can step either front-left or back-left because he has the option to decide where to go.

Leaders, it's always best to start a move after completing a basic (left then right), but it's not an absolute. If you wanted to start back-right, for instance, you could do so after doing the left part of your side basic, but it might confuse you up front if you mix the moves up too much.

Until you're comfortable, you might want to stay with the structure of doing everything in sets of two.

To practice all of what you know at this point, turn on your favorite song and assume the position (the four connection points and your ready position). Leaders, you'll want to start out doing the basics a time or two or three or four, and then, when you're ready, try to go either front-left after completing a basic or back-left and see what happens.

Immediately thereafter, try to return to where you started, and then either go into your default basics again or go directly into another direction (either the same one you just did or the opposite directions). Play with it by trying different directions over and over until both you and your partner feel good about it, and don't be afraid to make mistakes. Mistakes will happen, and feet will probably be stepped on. It's okay! In fact, it's perfectly normal. Just be courteous and respectful when it happens, and try to laugh it off as much as possible. The more fun you have with it, the better your chances of continuing the practice and of practicing what's right.

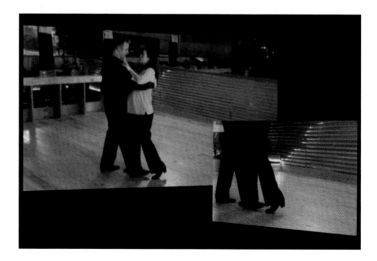

Left and Right Turns

H ERE'S THE PART where you get to start moving around in different directions. No longer will you have stay one-dimensional by just going back and forth and frontward and backward. You'll now get a chance to move in a circle you'll create, either to the left or to the right. Remember, the moves are called out for the leaders, so if it's called a left turn, the leader will be turning to the left, and if it's a right turn, the leader will be turning off to the right. It's important for the followers not to get caught up in the names, or else they'll be thinking about directions and not following them. We'll start out with the left turns because they're typically a bit more difficult than the right ones.

Left Turns

The left turns will enable you to add movement and change your direction. This move is called a *left turn* because you will be turning to the leader's left.

For the Leaders

Leaders, you'll want to start with one basic left to right, and then stop once you get to your ready position. On your next basic, you'll step back on the first count into an extended third foot position, which means although you're stepping back, you'll be stepping back and turning your left foot to face a new direction. Try to keep the step fairly small, maybe eight inches or less from the back of your right foot. You'll then tap your right foot together on two (first foot position with your weight still on your left foot), and then step right with your right foot on three (back to the second foot position), and then tap your left foot together on four (back to the first foot position), which brings you back into the ready position to start a new direction. At the right is the visual depiction of your steps.

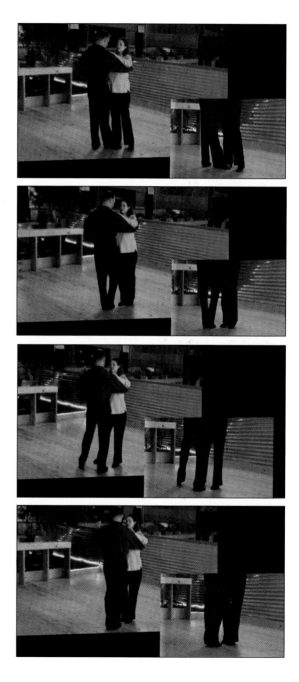

For the Followers

Followers, your steps are the exact opposite on this one. You're going to step front-right on the first count, but you'll do so a bit differently—your foot will end up facing your partner, rather than facing away from him. Take a look at the first figure at the right to get a visual of this. Then, you'll tap your left foot together on two (first foot position with your weight still on your right foot), and then step left with your left foot on three, and then tap your right foot together on four (back to the first foot position), which brings you back into the ready position to start a new direction.

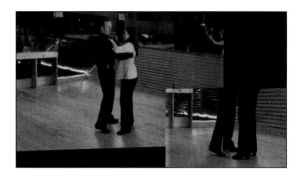

Right Turns

Another movement-maker, right turns will allow you to "unwind" from your left-hand turns. Like left turns, the name *right turn* is assigned because you will be turning to the leader's right.

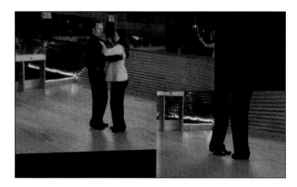

For the Leaders

The right turn starts out a bit differently than the other steps that we've done to this point. On this one, leaders, you'll want to start from a ready position and do a half of a basic, which means you'll step left with your left foot (into the second foot position) on the first count. On count two, you'll bring your right foot together and touch (first foot position). The first two steps here are essentially the first half of a basic. The next two steps are where all the action happens for the right turns, so buckle up and hold on tight. Now that your weight is on your left foot and your right foot is free to step, you're going to step off to the right into an extended third foot position (see the third figure at the right), where you'll step directly between your partner's two feet if this is done correctly. Count four on this one is simply bringing your left foot together (back to the first foot position in a new direction) and tapping, which brings you back into the ready position so you can start a new move.

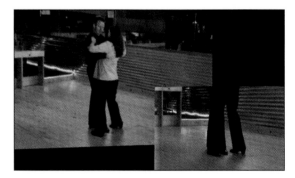

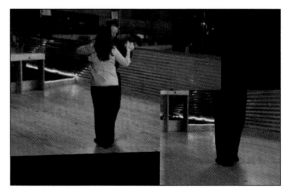

Leaders, make sure you shift your entire frame to the right when you're placing your partner where she needs to go. Connection point 2 is used the most for this one, as you'll feel like you're pulling your partner into place to get her to step where she needs to.

For the Followers

Just like all the other steps thus far, the followers' steps are the exact opposite on this one. The first two counts are the same as your regular basics (step right with your right and then touch with your left). Through this point, you should feel nothing different in the lead, as it feels like you're doing the basics. As you go to step with your left for count three, you should feel like you're being pulled forward and to the right, which will force your body into turning toward your partner as you step. You'll essentially be cutting the corner and doing about a quarter turn to the right as you step forward with your left. At the end of count three, you should be facing your partner with your weight on your left foot, and your partner's right foot should be just to the right of your left. (His right foot is supposed to be in between your two feet.) Count four should be your normal count four, as you'll bring your right foot together (into the first foot position) and tap. At this point, you'll be back to the ready position and ready to start the next move.

Fun Drills to Put It All Together

FOLLOWING ARE a number of drills set up specifically for you to practice what you've learned. Instead of just picturing yourself slow dancing, this is where you'll put it all together and dance it for yourself. Try to go through each one of the drills because they focus on different moves, leads, and thinking patterns. At this point, you should feel confident enough to take your slow dance with you just about anywhere to show it off.

Drill 1: Normal, Close, and Really Close (Three Different Distances)

Set up in your ready position and four connection points and do the basics a couple of times. Stop and set up again, but this time you should cut the space between you and your partner in half and try a few more basics. Then, stop a second time and reposition yourself again. This time, you should almost be touching with your bodies. You'll notice that the connection points will have to change slightly to account for the close quarters, but that you can still do the leading and following. There will be an appropriate time for each of these distances, and you'll get to pick it. Try them out and test the different moves at each distance, as shown in the images on this page.

Followers, as your stance gets closer, your connection point 4 becomes more and more important. A quick and sneaky way to maintain your part of the dance frame when extremely close to your leader is to make sure you are offset to the left. This will also help your neck if you are shorter than your partner. If your partner is to your right, you can press up against his shoulder blade and still look him in the eye without getting a kink in your neck from looking up at him from the side rather than directly head-on.

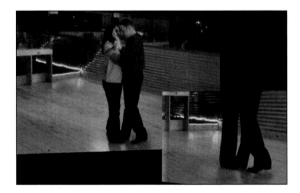

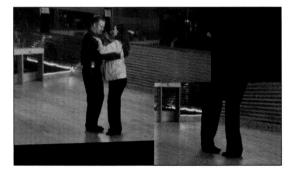

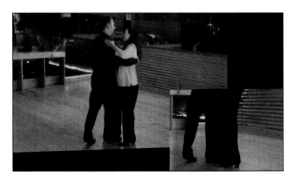

Drill 2: Slow, Medium, and Fast (Three Different Speeds)

Turn on the radio and test out a few different songs. Try to dance to a few different speeds so you'll know what you're most comfortable with. Some songs will be so slow that you feel like you're dragging, and other songs you considered slow will feel more like a swing once you start dancing to the beat. It's best to test the different song speeds at home so you'll get a good feel for them prior to being out in front of others. For the really slow songs, you'll see that it takes quite a bit more control than for the faster ones, and the ones in the middle will feel very comfortable. Go ahead; give a few songs a try.

Drill 3: The Basics, Front and Back

Here, you'll go back and work on just the basics, but you'll do them left and right, and then front and back, and in non-repeating patterns that cover each step. Start with a few basics, then do them front and back, then a basic or two, then back and front, and so on. This drill will reinforce the leaders' ability to change direction and the followers' ability to follow. Practice these steps until both partners are comfortable moving in each direction. You can combine this drill with Drill 1 or 2.

Drill 4: Left and Right Turns

Start with a couple of basics and then do two or three left turns. Then, after a basic or two, do a few right turns until you're comfortable. After you've done each of them individually, start combining them—do a left turn, then a right, then a left, then two right turns, and so on, just to mix it up and test the lead.

Drill 5: Putting It All Together

Here, you'll take your first real shot at putting it all together. Go through each of the moves one time in a very controlled manner. First the basics, then the front and back basics, then the combination of the two, then the left turns, then the right turns, and so on. Once you've gone through them once, try to put your own spin on things. Leaders, try to dance through each of the moves, but put them in a different order so the follower cannot predict what's coming up. This will help with your lead and also with her follow. Try them many different ways until you're both comfortable.

Drill 6: Testing the Lead

Leaders, this is where it gets fun and interesting. Go ahead and drop connection point 1 and use only connection points 2, 3, and 4. You're now going to lead your partner through all of the different moves, but you're going to do it without your left hand. First, just work on the basics. Do a few left and right and focus on using your right hand as a guide for both directions. Then, add in the front and back basics combined with the left and right basics. Now you should start to feel like you're really taking hold here. It's about to get interesting. When you're comfortable with the basics in all directions, you get to try the left and right turns. Start with the left turns and see how it goes. Try not to be forceful (remember, this is a smooth dance) as you place your partner in front of you over and over. Then, change direction and go the other way for the right turns. This one should feel a bit easier for you if you have the right control. After you've done each direction, start looking to combine all the moves together and try to dance an entire song.

Hot Tips for Slow Dancing

NOW THAT YOU'VE HAD a chance to go through the slow dancing, it's time to reinforce a few traits and give you a few pointers on how to make you and your partner look good. Take a look at the following tips and try to work them into your dance.

▶ Slow dancing with someone does not automatically give you the right to hang all over that person or press your body directly up against him or her. Respect your partner and use the connection points to your advantage. However, if the situation allows for extremely close connections, then don't be afraid to use them.

▶ Dancing together at the same speed is more important than dancing to the speed of the song. Followers, take note. If the leader is dancing slower or faster than the song, try to follow along with his speed rather than the speed of the song. Everyone will notice if the two of you are dancing to two different beats, but you might be the only one who notices you are offbeat if you are dancing in unison.

▶ Avoid the temptation to sing along to every word of the song playing. There might be times when you'll want to emphasize a phrase or two just for fun, but let the singing stay in the voices of the recorded artists.

▶ For the sake of your partner and everyone watching, don't let your hands slide down onto your partner's rear end. As tempting as this might be, most people are uncomfortable with this position, and almost everyone who's watching will find it extremely tacky. Most importantly, whatever you do, don't attempt this "connection point" with a stranger.

▶ As a leader, be careful with dipping your partner. If you've never practiced a dip or if you don't know how to do one, trying it out during your dance is not recommended. If you're going to dip your partner, do it gently and with control. It's not uncommon for both partners to end up on the floor on a poorly executed dip. Know your limitations.

▶ Enjoy your dance. Above all else, try to enjoy the moment while you're doing the slow dance. Take in the surroundings, the music, the atmosphere, the feelings, and so on. Let your body relax and go on cruise control, especially if you're comfortable with the leading and following drills from earlier in the chapter. Don't overdo it, and your partner will want to do it again, and again, and again....

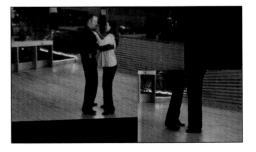

Review and Next Steps for Your Slow Dance

Congratulations! You've made it through your first dance. You're now ready to heat up the dance floor with a smooth and romantic slow dance. To review everything you've gone through, we've made a quick little checklist for you. See whether you can go right down it and put yourself in each position and move without much thought. Start with number 1 and go straight through.

Review

1. Ladies are always right! Ladies, put your weight on your left foot so you can be ready to start with your right. (This is what's called your *ready position.*)

2. Guys always get what's left. Guys, put your weight on your right foot so you can be ready to start with your left. (This is what's called your *ready position.*)

3. All four connection points are used in the basics of the slow dance.

4. The slow-dance basic consists of four counts (step, touch, step, touch).

5. The basics can be done in almost any direction (front, back, left, right, front-left, back-right, back-left, and front-right).

6. Always go back to the basics when you're not sure of what else to do. The basics should be your default movement during the slow dance, whether the music is slow or fast and regardless of how close in distance you are to your partner.

7. Left turns start on count one with the leader stepping back with his left.

8. Right turns start on count three with the leader doing a half basic with his left, and then stepping off to the right.

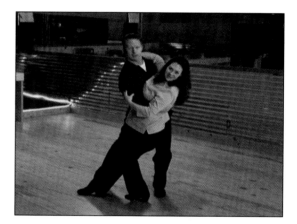

Next Steps

When you're comfortable with the slow dance that you've gone through, you might want to take it a bit further. There are many more facets of the dance that you can easily add into your repertoire. Underarm turns (arches), momentum turns, dips, and leans can all easily be added into your dance once you're comfortable with the basics. Take it one step at a time and have fun while you learn. The slow dance is one of the most versatile and romantic dances if done correctly.

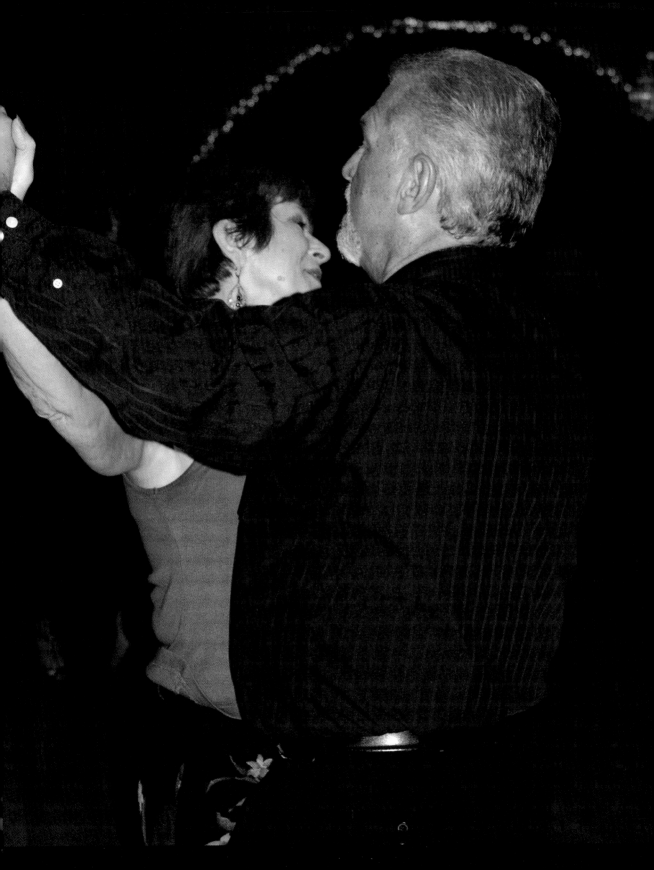

4

Picture Yourself

Dancing
the Waltz

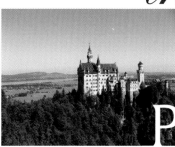

© istockphoto.com/Dainis Derics

PICTURE YOURSELF waltzing around the room to the melodic strains of one of the masterpiece compositions of Johann Strauss. The other couples around you are following the ebb and flow of the same lilting melody as all parties rotate and circulate around the floor. As the vivacious music fills the room, men's coattails lift and ladies' dresses swirl as the couples rise and fall with the energetic music. Clear the canvas in your mind, and now picture yourself gliding gracefully around the floor to either a country-western or contemporary love song written in three-quarter time. You aren't moving at nearly the same pace as you were in the first image, but this dance is truly one of romance. As you rise and fall with the highs and lows in the musical line while progressing around the dance floor, a sensation of floating is created, much like the euphoria of romance. In the moments after the music fades, this feeling lingers in the atmosphere like a fine perfume. In both images the music evokes images of yesteryear, but the exhilaration associated with the momentum created during the waltz is as fresh today as it was in the eighteenth and nineteenth centuries.

The Six Ws of Waltz

THE WALTZ is considered the parent of all social ballroom dances. It is one of the oldest social dances, with a rich history marked by controversy and wild popularity.

Who Popularized the Waltz?

Waltz as we know it today, with the closed dance position and independently dancing couples, was popularized in the high-society circles of Europe. The French especially adopted the waltz with alacrity. The waltz was created to accompany a very specific type of music that gained enormous popularity through the work of various period composers, the frontrunners being Joseph Lanner and Johann Strauss. As with almost all things European, the waltz made its way across the Atlantic and became a firmly grounded bastion of American ballroom dancing.

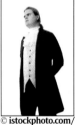

© istockphoto.com/
Amanda Rohde

What Is the Waltz?

The waltz is a progressive dance that is done in three-quarter time, meaning that there is a six-count basic and the music that the waltz accompanies has three beats per measure. If you were to hum along with a waltz, you would feel the underlying bum-buh-buh, bum-buh-buh.

There are two types of waltz, Viennese and the modern waltz. The Viennese waltz is marked by an extremely quick tempo, while the modern waltz has a more romantic look to the slower waltz songs. However, all forms of waltz are marked by a characteristic rise and fall that matches the musical percussive emphasis on the first beat of every measure.

A *progressive dance* describes any dance where the partners dance around the perimeter of the dance floor in a counterclockwise direction. All of the turns, spins, and other moves are done while the partners are progressing around the floor.

Where Did the Waltz Originate and Where Is It Typically Done?

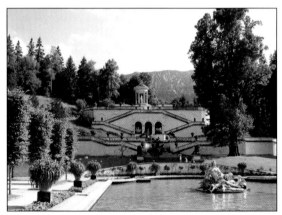

© istockphoto.com/Dainis Derics

The waltz originated in the folk dances of the Bavarian and Austrian Alps, but truly gained popularity in the ballrooms of the Austrian court. From Austria, the music and the dance spread across Europe. As the popularity of the waltz and the associated music grew, the dance traveled across the Atlantic Ocean to the United States.

As a parent dance for all of the modern ballroom dances, waltz is most frequently done in ballrooms. However, because the waltz can be danced to any song that has three-quarter timing, a slow version of the waltz is also seen in the country-western world. The waltz is also a popular choice for a choreographed first dance at a wedding, though music choice is much more limited than it is with the other contemporary ballroom dances. The waltz is also a staple at such events as Quinceañera, debuts, and other formal coming-of-age social events.

When Did the Waltz Become Popular and When Is the Right Time to Waltz?

The exact birth date of the waltz is unknown, but it is firmly established that contredanse versions of the waltz were performed in European high society to three-quarter time music in the mid-eighteenth century.

The version of the waltz that we dance today, with couples dancing independently in closed dance positions, emerged toward the end of the eighteenth century. For the early years of the nineteenth century, the waltz was, for the most part, contained to continental European and then English high society. The waltz was introduced to the New World in 1834 at an exhibition in Boston, Massachusetts. The waltz gained a firm foothold in American social dancing and paved the way for the remainder of the ballroom dances.

The right time to waltz can be described as any time you hear an appropriate song. Because there are two established and accepted tempos for the waltz, Viennese and modern, if the timing of the music is three-quarter time, there could potentially be immeasurable opportunities to dance the waltz in an evening. The waltz can be an exhilarating and

Contredanse **is a form of choreographed group dancing. Contemporary square dancing is a modern-day contredanse. Although the dancers are divided into couples, the couples dance together to form the overall dance.**

upbeat breath-stealer of a Viennese waltz or a soft, slow, and lilting modern waltz, depending on the song. This is why historically, during the waltz's heyday, an evening at the ballroom would be 90-percent waltz and 10-percent everything else.

Why Is the Waltz Danced?

Depending on the tempo, the waltz is danced for several reasons. The Viennese waltz is an exuberant celebration of your dance partner, the song, and life in general in its very rapid tempo and quick turns and upbeat music. The modern waltz is a more stately and formal exhibition of the dance partner as you travel around the floor. In its adolescence and prime, all versions of the waltz were considered very risqué and intimate, but the waltz of today is considered a very romantic, yet formal dance.

What Kind of Attire Should Be Worn?

There is no dress code or standard apparel for the waltz; however, you will typically see the waltz and dance the waltz at formal occasions, so dress to the occasion. The major exception to this rule is the country-western waltz, which is done to songs as a part of a dance set along with two-step, West coast swing, East coast swing, and occasionally cha-cha at country nightclubs. At a country-western nightclub, you would be more appropriately dressed in informal attire.

Visualize the Waltz

BEFORE STARTING THE LESSON PLAN for each dance, it's recommended you take a few minutes or so to watch the accompanying DVD and view the current section. In this case, you'll be watching the waltz segment to allow your mind's eye to start processing ideas on how to get your body to do what you're watching. Visualizing the waltz will give you a good feel for what you're about to learn and will make the transition into reality that much easier.

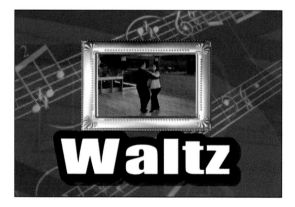

It's best if you watch the waltz section one time through without trying to do any of it. Just give your mind a chance to absorb the material so it's somewhat familiar to you when you hit replay to start the section over again. Watch how the dancers move, think about the words that are used, and picture yourself dancing the waltz.

The second time you watch the DVD, it's recommended that you take notes. Jot down the important parts of the waltz so you can engage other parts of the kinesthetic learning prior to getting up and dancing along. Write down what the connection points are, what the basic steps are called,

how many counts are in a basic, how to align with your partner, and so on. Also, write down any questions that you might have about the waltz. There's a good chance you will find the answer later in this chapter, and if it's something you're already pondering, you'll be sure to remember the answer.

You'll find that by time you get ready to stand up and try the waltz with the DVD, the dancing won't be nearly as overwhelming. Writing down the key concepts will allow you to get a jumpstart on the rest of this chapter. You'll find that after you get up and try it, you'll probably have more questions. As this chapter goes on, the steps will be broken out with screenshots from the DVD, pointers will be given on where you should be during different parts of the dance, and frequently asked questions will be addressed that should satisfy most (if not all) of your questions and then some.

The third time you view the DVD, go ahead and dance along with it. See how far you can make it just by watching and trying. You'll probably find that one of the two of you is able to pick up and understand the material more quickly than the other.

> **Just remember, everyone learns at different paces. Be cognizant of this as you're learning with your partner. One of you might pick up certain aspects of the dance quicker than the other, and that's okay. Try to be patient and wait for the other person to grasp the material, and then move on.**

Now take a look at the rest of these pictures. All of them are taken of couples dancing the waltz. Some are formal, some are very informal, but they're all doing the same steps. See whether you can visualize yourself waltzing (the dance you just watched over and over) in all these different settings. Then, picture yourself waltzing at upcoming events or at local venues where you and your partner can go out. Where will you go out dancing after you learn the waltz? Start thinking of the possibilities.

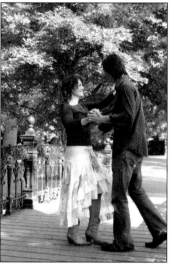

© istockphoto.com/Simone van den Berg

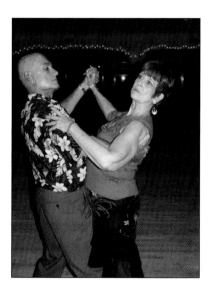

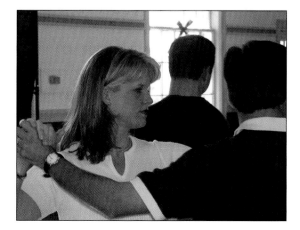

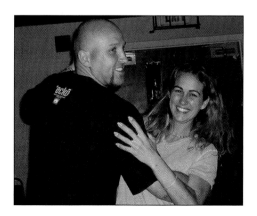

Waltz Basics

THE WALTZ is considered by many to be the mother of today's couples dances. Once known for its seductiveness and immoral connotations due to the tight closed position and rapid and constant turning, the waltz today is known for its distinctive rise and fall look because it is elegant, smooth, and beautiful on the dance floor.

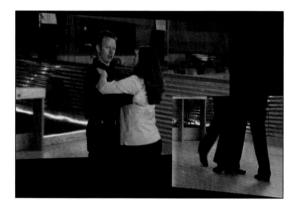

> *Rise and fall* is a continuous change of body elevation combining an upward shift of your body and then a slow and even lowering. The *rise* can be done with the feet or ankles, and sometimes the lengthening of the torso, and the *fall* is done by compressing into bent or flexed knees and/or ankles.

As previously mentioned, the waltz is danced to three-quarter timing, which means the number of songs to which you can practice is quite limited if you're just turning on your radio or pulling out your CD or MP3 collection. It might be best to do

a search online for "waltz music" and find a few songs from whatever genre of music is your favorite and then practice along. At the very least, try to understand and get familiar with the timing in order to recognize the dance when the opportunity arises. Before you begin the waltz, let's recap the two most important rules:

1. Ladies are always right! Ladies, put your weight on your left foot so you can be ready to start with your right. (This is what's called your *ready position*.)

2. Guys always get what's left. Guys, put your weight on your right foot so you can be ready to start with your left. (This is what's called your *ready position*.)

The Six-Count Basic (Box Step)

The six-count basic of waltz is made up of one box step, or two sets of half boxes and the distinctive rise and fall. Each step in the waltz contains the same amount of time—one beat—even though the strongest accent is on counts 1 and 4. Waltz, in layman's terms, is said out loud like this:

Step, side, together,

Step, side, together

If you're more mathematically inclined and like to use numbers, it's counted like this:

One, two, three,

Four, five, six

For the correct rise and fall look and feel, you'll want to let your body lower slightly on the first count, rise on the second count, and start to lower again on the third. (The same holds true for counts 4, 5, and 6.) It's a continuous, yet soft, up and down motion that should appear effortless and flowing.

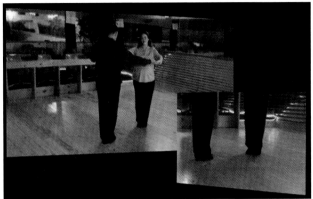

To try the waltz basics in place, assume foot position 1 and be in your respective ready position. Next, you'll want to simply take six steps in a row, changing weight each time and counting them aloud (either 1-2-3, 4-5-6 or step, step, together, step, step, together). Doing this a few times should get you familiar with the timing and the changing of weight. At the end of every six counts, you should be back in your ready position, which means you and your partner will be on opposite feet the entire time, even when you stop.

Mirroring

When you're comfortable with the basics in place, go ahead and move into the next steps, which will allow you to do the basics of waltz without having to worry about anything but the footwork. For learning your individual steps the first time, stand directly in front of each other. Try facing each other as shown in the figure on the right, but be about two to five feet away from your partner in a mirrored position. It often helps if you're able to see the opposite steps, if for no other reason than to validate your own. Below the mirroring is demonstrated in a two-hand hold rather than open dance position. If you find the hand connection distracting at this point, do not hesitate to drop the connection points and focus on your feet exclusively.

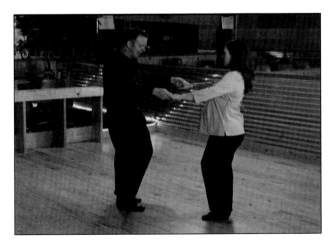

1. (Step 1) From a ready position, leaders will step straight forward with their left foot (fourth foot position) and followers will step straight back with their right foot (also a fourth foot position), with each partner changing weight to the foot that was moving by the end of step or count 1.

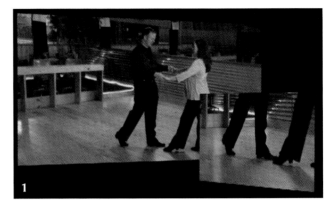

2. (Step 2) Leaders, step with your right foot to the right side about shoulder-width apart from your left foot (second foot position). Followers, step with your left to your left side about shoulder-width apart from your right foot (second foot position). Again, make sure to change weight to the foot that was moving during this step.

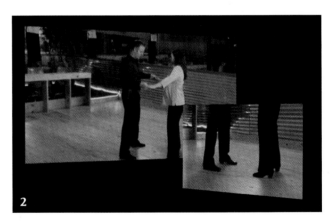

3. (Step 3) Leaders, step with your left foot to the right side, bringing your feet together into the first foot position. Followers, step with your right to your left side, bringing your feet together into the first foot position. Make sure you change weight to the foot that was just moving; this is a step where many errors are made due to not changing weight.

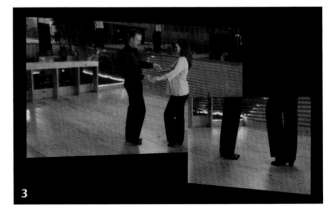

4. (Step 4) From a reverse ready position, leaders will step straight back with their right foot (fourth foot position) and followers will step straight forward with their left foot (also a fourth foot position), with each partner changing weight to the foot that was moving during step or count 4.

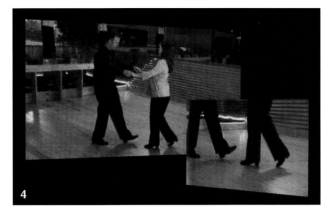

5. (Step 5) Leaders, step with your left foot to the left side about shoulder-width apart from your right foot (second foot position). Followers, step with your right to your right side about shoulder-width apart from your left foot (second foot position). Again, on this one, both partners change weight to the foot that was moving during this step.

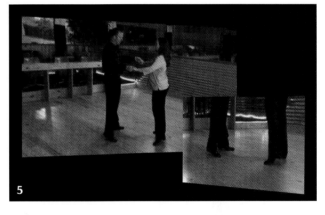

6. (Step 6) Leaders, step with your right foot to the left side, bringing your feet together into the first foot position (and subsequently, the ready position). Followers, step with your left to your right side, bringing your feet together into the first foot position (or ready position) also. Make sure you change weight to the foot that was just moving; this is another step where many errors are made due to not changing weight.

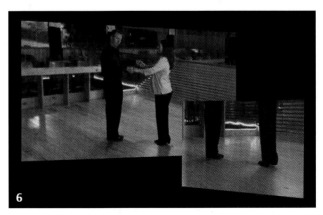

A *reverse ready position* is the exact opposite of your ready position. For example, if your weight is normally on your left foot for your ready position, this time it would be on your right.

Now that you're able to do a complete box step, go ahead and practice what you just learned with music. It'll be the last thing you try before putting it all together. Leaders, count out loud to give the follower a chance to match you step for step when you start. The leader should say "4-5-6" and then step with his left foot.

> **If either partner gets on the "wrong foot" during the exercise, just stop, laugh, and start up again after the leader counts it off…4-5-6 and you're back dancing again.**

Practice until you're both comfortable with the steps and the answers to each of the following questions.

> ▶ **Just before count 1, should you be in your ready position or reverse ready position?**
>
> ▶ **Are there any steps that you'll take in a six-count basic that do not include a change of weight?**
>
> ▶ **What are the foot positions used for steps 1 and 4, 2 and 5, and 3 and 6, respectively?**

The Six-Count Basic as a Couple

Now that you're both experts on doing the basics on your own in a made-up box, it's time to try them together. Hopefully you completed the previous exercise and didn't just skip right to the dancing. If you skipped right to the dancing and didn't practice it on your own, you might have a tough time figuring out where any problems are if they arise. Practicing before coming together is a critical building block; the confidence each partner brings makes it much easier because you'll both have high expectations. As said many times in this book, social dancing is probably close to 25-percent skill and 75-percent attitude, so let's keep up the good work and high spirits.

Your toolkit for the waltz basics includes:

> ▶ **Foot position 1 (ready position and counts 3 and 6 of the basic)**
>
> ▶ **Foot position 2 (counts 2 and 5 of the basic)**
>
> ▶ **Foot position 4 (counts 1 and 4 of the basic)**
>
> ▶ **Connection points 1–4 (all will be used here in the basic)**
>
> ▶ **Six-count basic (essential for the waltz to work)**

Okay, now get into position and start your waltz. The first thing you want to do is get into your dance position with your partner (use all four connection points), have your feet offset, and be in your ready position. Leaders, go ahead and give your countdown (4-5-6) and move forward with your left and then to your right with your right, then bring your left foot together with your right (halfway there). Now, step back with your right, step side with your left, and bring your right foot together with your left in the ready position. Now, just repeat it over and over. Okay, you're doing the basics now. . . . One, two, three, four, five, six, one, two, three, four, five, six. . .excellent!

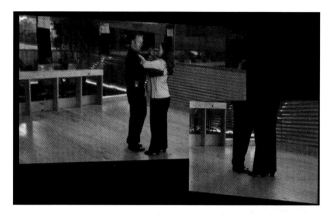

Now, let's make this one a bit more interesting. This time when you go to try it, the leaders should actually lead it. By leading, we're not talking about verbal leads; we're talking about through the body. Leaders, when you're ready, see whether you can put this together and make it work. You have four connection points that you'll use here to help you out. The two most important ones to start the waltz with are connection points 2 and 4. Leaders, your upper body must be in synch with your lower body on this one because you'll need to drive toward your partner, then take her to the side, then move away from your partner, and then to the side. A simultaneous and deliberate movement of both your feet and your torso in equal force forward, then to the right, then back, then to your left will leave your partner without wonder.

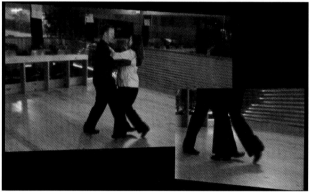

Did it work? If so, you did each of the following (you should aim for at least three of the four):

- ▶ **You successfully completed the six-count basic (a whole box step).**
- ▶ **You both changed weight six times during the basic.**
- ▶ **You managed to keep her directly in front of you.**
- ▶ **You kept a smile on her face or caused one.**

To recap on this one, there are several different leads going on during the waltz basic. The follower should be able to initially feel the leader coming directly toward her with connection points 1 and 4, then immediately thereafter feel all four connection points take her directly to the left. Followers, there should be no question as to what direction your body should be moving in, and your feet should come together nicely by count 3 with enough freedom to be able to step down onto your right foot. On count 4, followers, you should feel that you're as well connected as if you were on a ride at a theme park with braces all around you for support as you step forward with your left foot and the leader steps back with his right. The fifth count will bring both partners to the side again as you both softly prepare for the sixth and final step, a closure to the basic where it will all start up again from your ready position. Success is marked when everything is working together and both partners are moving effortlessly with one another.

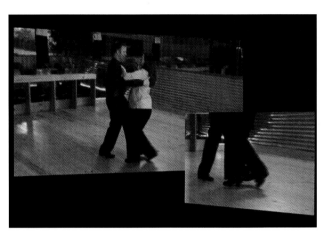

For the Followers

Followers, this next part is the same as it is in any dance and might be difficult to grasp because you want to help, but try your best. If the leader isn't perfectly clear on the lead (in other words, the motion or the guidance), don't move! Now, don't be stubborn and just stand there, but if the lead isn't nearly perfect, make him improve it. Focus on the problem if there is one. There shouldn't be much of an argument here—either you feel it and it's enough or you don't. The only major thing you need to concentrate on here is being in good frame and sitting slightly back into connection point 2.

For the Leaders

Leaders, you're up again. We continue to emphasize the following point throughout this text, so please, once again, take note. If you give a lady a choice (on the dance floor), she'll take it! If you leave the door open for interpretation, you never know what you'll end up with. Nothing personal here, ladies; it'd be the same if you were leading. Okay leaders, take your partner in your arms in closed dance position (with the four connection points, of course) and try the basics again. Try them over and over and practice the leads going forward and then to the side, then back and then to the other side. Have your follower close her eyes and see whether she can follow what you're doing. If you're leading correctly, your partner will match your speed and do exactly what your body tells her to do. If the follower is having difficulty (other than not understanding the basic footwork of the waltz basic), there's a better than 90-percent chance it has something to do with the lead.

The Turning Box Step (Left Turns)

Now that you're both experts on doing the basics front to back and side to side, you'll find that you might soon get bored, if you haven't already. What you'll do now is move not only in a box pattern, but also off at diagonals as you turn around the dance floor. (And yes, you'll use most of your eight directional possibilities on these as well.) The step-by-step guide is broken out for leaders and followers separately, but you should both try to learn the footwork for both partners to give you a better perspective of what's happening with your partner. Start with doing one basic, then stop in your ready position.

For the Leaders: Part 1

Leaders, you're going to step front-left on the first count (extended third foot position), but as you do so you'll want to step all the way onto your left foot and start turning your body to the left as well (approximately one-eighth of a turn at this point). On the second step, you'll continue your forward motion while you're turning and do another eighth turn to the left as your right foot will now step to the right into the second foot position. You've now turned a quarter turn to the left from where you started (an eighth turn on the first step and an eighth on the second). Count 3 is easy because it's the same as what you've been doing up to this point. Simply bring your feet together into the first foot position and change weight onto your left foot. Before you get too much further, go back and practice just this part until you have it. Each time you start, you should be in your ready position and then end up a quarter turn to your left at the end of the first three counts. At the right is the visual depiction of your steps.

Part 1

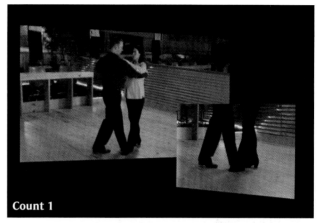

Count 1

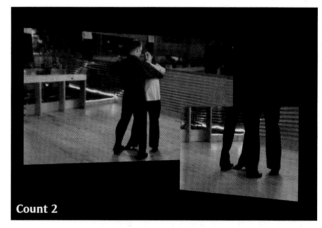

Count 2

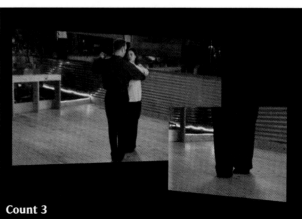

Count 3

For the Followers: Part 1

Followers, your steps are the exact opposite on this one. You're going to step back-right on the first count as you also do a eighth turn to the left. (This might feel a bit more natural when the guy is actually leading it.) On the second count, you'll continue your motion and do another eighth turn to the left while your left foot steps into the second foot position. By the end of the second step, you should have made a quarter turn back to your left from where you started, and you should be prepared to step with your right foot to bring it together. On count 3, your right foot will come together with your left in the first foot position, and you'll then place weight on it. Practice the first three counts several times until you're comfortable, and then move onto Part 2. Just remember, each time you go to start, get into your ready position.

For the Leaders: Part 2

You'll now add on to what you just learned in Part 1. You've just gone through the first three steps, and you're on your left foot and ready to start with your right (also known as the reverse ready position). With your right foot, you'll now step back-right on the fourth count as you do another eighth turn to the left. Place your weight onto your right foot as your momentum is moving both backward and to your left. On the fifth count, you'll do another eighth turn to your left as you step with your left foot to the left into the second foot position. Make sure your weight is on your left foot. On the sixth and final count, you'll step with your right foot into the first foot position, which brings you back into the ready position to start another basic or another turn. At the right is the visual depiction of the steps.

Part 2

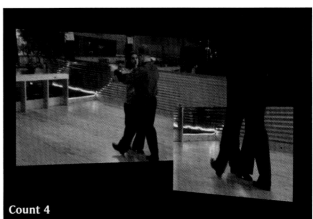

Count 4

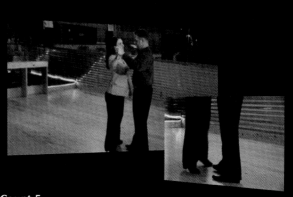

Count 5

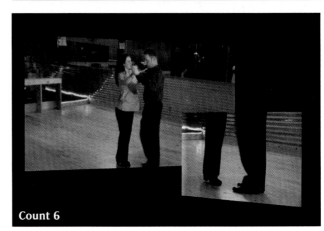

Count 6

For the Followers: Part 2

Followers, your steps are the exact opposite on this one. Remember, you've just gone through and done the first three steps, and you're now on your right foot, ready to start with your left. You're going to step front-left with your left foot on the fourth count as you start to turn to your left (again, approximately an eighth of a turn). Your momentum is moving forward and rotating to the left. You'll continue your momentum and do another eighth of a turn to the left as you step out to the right into the second foot position with your right foot. Make sure your weight is down and changed to your right foot before count 6. On 6, you'll step your left foot together with your right foot into the first foot position and change weight, which will bring you back into the ready position to start again.

New Dimension to the Lead

When you were just doing the box step in the six-count basic, the lead was fairly cut and dried as you went forward, then to the side, then back, then to the side, and so on. Now you'll add the dimension of turning your partner as you step forward and backward, and not everything will work the first time you try it. The easiest way to get through the turning box is to think of it as a continuous revolution and not so much as a little turn here and a little turn there. When you start each half of the turn, don't stop until counts 3 and then 6. Work your way through each one so that you're thinking, "Turn, turn, together, turn, turn, together," and so on. You'll practice it more here in just a minute.

Practicing the Turning Box Step

To practice the turning box step, it's best to first try it together, without any connection points. Give yourselves about two feet or so of distance between you, and then walk through the six counts a couple of times. You'll get a better sense of how it all comes together and where each of you should be at any given point. When you're comfortable doing it on your own, set up in your closed dance position and give it a shot. Leaders, again, on this one you'll be focusing on moving toward your partner and on the continuous turn. Keep your frame where it needs to be and your lead clear and constant, and there shouldn't be any problems. You'll want to practice this step over and over, but don't fall into the temptation of doing the turns so many times without a basic in the middle that neither of you can see straight. As soon as you're able to deliberately do the turning box step, you can move on to the next part, where you'll be mixing it up with the basics and then doing parts of the turn individually to give you a few more patterns to work with.

Mixing up the Directions for Practice

Leaders, you now get to put a few of these pieces together to test out your lead. The steps you can mix up and execute in almost any order include:

- ▶ **The box step**
- ▶ **Quarter turn left (turning box with left foot on counts 1, 2, and 3)**
- ▶ **Quarter turn left (turning box with right foot on counts 4, 5, and 6)**
- ▶ **Continuous turning box (quarter turn left on 1, 2, and 3, then quarter turn left on 4, 5, and 6)**

The box step is what you should consider your default basic. If at any time during the dance the leader cannot think of anything else to do or just wants to take it easy for a moment, these are the steps that should be done. Then, at any point thereafter, the leader can choose what the next step is going to be. With four options to choose from (see the preceding bulleted list), the leader can now start to make some fun decisions.

Leaders, you now get to mix and match the four different options here. First, try to put them all together. Do a few basics, then add in just the first left turn, then do a few basics, then add in the second left turn, then put them both together with the continuous box. This will be a true test of your ability to differentiate between a turn and a regular basic. Spend some time here to really make it right as you work through each of these options. Followers, do your best to only move and turn as the lead guides you. If need be, don't be afraid to close your eyes and just let him take you along for the ride. It sometimes works out better for both parties because he might not be as intimidated by your glare in response to each mistake. Just give it some time until it feels right, then move on to the next step.

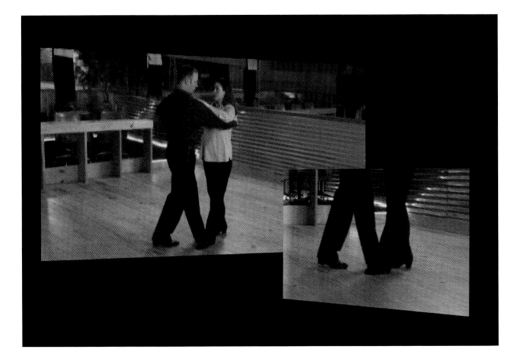

Progressive Basics

ANOTHER WAY of doing the six basic steps is to do them in a progressive manner, where each step will pass the other and you'll move around the dance floor. As with any other progressive movements in couples dancing, you'll want to move counterclockwise around the dance floor and stay toward the outside of the floor. To do the progressive basics, you'll do the same six counts where there are six changes of weight, and you'll still have the same rise and fall that you had with the box step. It's more common on a country dance floor to see the progressive basics of the waltz than in a ballroom, but the moves are inter-changeable and look good in either setting.

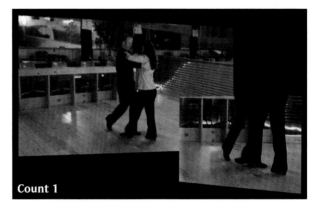

Count 1

For the Leaders

Leaders, you're going to step forward on the first count (fourth foot position), directly toward your partner in a driving motion. On the second step, you're going to continue your forward motion with-out deviation as your right foot will now step forward into the fourth foot position. Count 3 is a little differ-ent than what you've been doing up to this point because your feet will not come together; they'll just continue moving forward into the fourth foot posi-tion again as you change weight onto your left foot. Counts 4, 5, and 6 are identical because you'll just continue moving forward along the outside of the dance floor. To add in the rise and fall in the progres-sive basics, you'll want to step on count 1 in more of a driving motion (like an airplane on a runway), and then on the second step, you'll want to rise and you'll stay up through part of the third step and then fall (come down) as you complete the half basic. The sec-ond half of the basic is done the same way. At the right and on the next page is a visual depiction of both the leader's and the follower's footwork.

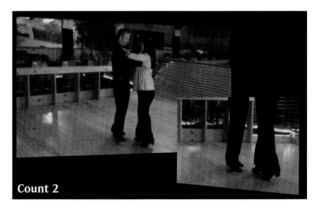

Count 2

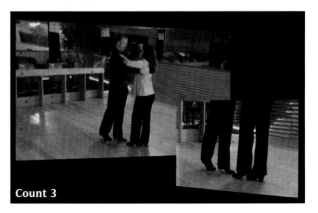

Count 3

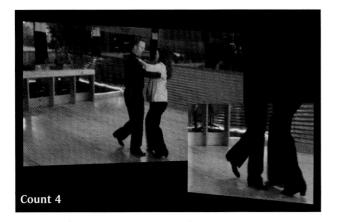

Count 4

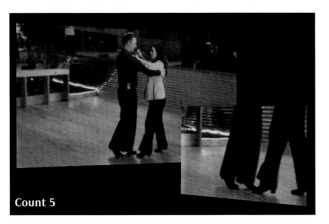

Count 5

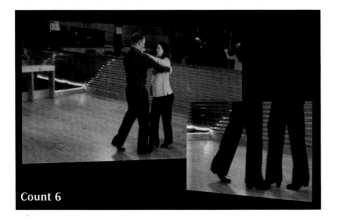

Count 6

For the Followers

Followers, your steps are the exact opposite on this one. You'll step backward on the first count (fourth foot position), directly away from your partner down the line of dance. On the second step, you'll continue your backward motion without deviation as your left foot will now step backward into the fourth foot position. Count 3 is a little different than what you've been doing up to this point because your feet will not come together; they'll just continue moving backward into the fourth foot position again as you change weight onto your right foot. Counts 4, 5, and 6 are identical as you continue moving backward along the outside of the dance floor. Just like the leaders, to add in the rise and fall in the progressive basics, you'll want to step on count 1 in more of a driving motion (like an airplane on a runway), then on the second step, you'll want to rise, and you'll stay up through part of the third step and then fall (come down) as you complete the half basic. The second half of the basic is done the same way.

Fun Drills to Put It All Together

FOLLOWING ARE a number of drills set up specifically for you to practice what you've learned. Instead of just picturing yourself doing the waltz, this is where you'll put it all together and dance it all for yourself. Try to go through each one of the drills because they focus on different moves, leads, and thinking patterns. By the end of these drills, you should feel confident enough to try your waltz out almost anywhere.

Drill 1: Dancing Solo

Set up in your ready position with your frame set for the four connection points and do the basics on your own without your partner. Have your partner watch and point out the things you're doing correctly. If there are areas of improvement, your partner should stop watching and attempt to do them alongside of you, and you can both work on them together. Then, once you're both satisfied, let the other demonstrate his or her steps, and you can watch and point out what's right. Finding the good in what your partner is doing is much more helpful than looking for what's wrong.

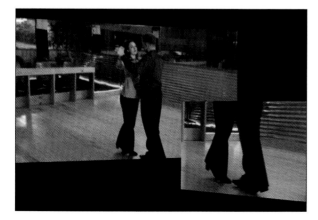

Drill 2: Slow, Medium, and Fast (Three Different Speeds)

Set up in your ready position, but this time with your partner, and test several different speeds of the waltz. You don't even need music to do this, just a leader who's willing to try it at his own pace, literally. When the leader is going very slowly, you'll see that it takes quite a bit more control than when it's faster, and the ones in the middle will feel very comfortable. If you have waltz music, go ahead and give a few songs a try.

Drill 3: Two of a Kind

Here, the leaders get to go through each of the moves that they learned in this section and try them one after another after another. Leaders, you'll do two of each move starting with the basic box step, then you'll do two sets of the left turns, then you'll do two progressive basics, then you'll repeat it. Followers, even though you know what's coming up here, try to let the leader lead you through each step.

Drill 4: Mixing and Matching

Here, you'll go back and incorporate everything you learned together into one drill. The leaders get to choose the pattern or the order of the moves as you work your way through the basic box step, the turning box (left turns), and also the progressive basics. The leader can mix and match as he best sees fit. For example, the leader can start off by doing a progressive basic, then a left turn, then another left turn, then a box step, then another left turn. The leader gets to choose, but is responsible for maintaining the flow of the dance and for keeping the follower on track.

Hot Tips for the Waltz

YOU SHOULD NOW have a good feel for what the waltz is all about. Following are a number of tips and pointers to help reinforce what you've learned.

▶ Waltz is an elegant dance that is best stylized by the dancers keeping their upper bodies and heads erect. Either partner looking down detracts from the look of the dance and also throws off the balance of the couple because the head is no longer aligned with the center point of balance.

▶ Rise and fall is an important part of the dance. On the first count your body should lower slightly, and then you should gradually come up on the second count and stay up through part of the third until you lower again to start the next three steps.

▶ Steps that are taken to the side in the waltz should not exceed the shoulder-width of the smaller partner.

▶ It's especially important in the waltz to maintain your frame and connection. Because the leader must be able to move in any given direction, all connection points must be working together, and both partners must be able to use them effectively.

▶ The basics in waltz are the most important steps. Do them well, and you'll be able to do almost anything out on the dance floor. Practice them until they become second nature to you.

▶ Having your feet offset to start the dance (the leader's right foot should be between the follower's two feet) is especially important because the leader's first step is toward his partner. If the leader is directly in front of his partner and his partner doesn't move, someone's getting stepped on. Also, having your feet offset enables both partners to be able to look over the shoulder of the person they're dancing with. This is especially important as you move around the dance floor because you need to be aware of your surroundings.

▶ The waltz should look as though it's flowing. If it looks or even feels like it's choppy, it probably is. There should be a continuous flow of movement, and it should never really come to a stop until the end of the dance. Work on putting "fluidity" into your waltz by using natural body movements rather than stiff-legged patterns that are memorized.

▶ Enjoy the dance. Above all else, try to enjoy the moment while you're dancing the waltz. Take in the surroundings, the music, the atmosphere, the feelings, and so on. Let your body relax and go on cruise control, especially if you're comfortable with the leading and following drills from earlier in the chapter. Don't overdo it, and your partner will crave more from you.

Review and Next Steps for Your Waltz

FANTASTIC! If you're starting from the beginning, you've now completed two dances. To ensure that you're comfortable and to do a final recap, we're going to run back through the major points of what you've learned. Go through each one and come back to this list as necessary for a quick review. Start at the beginning and work your way through each point.

Review

1. Ladies are always right! Ladies, put your weight on your left foot so you can be ready to start with your right. (In other words, get in your ready position.)

2. Guys always get what's left. Guys, put your weight on your right foot so you can be ready to start with your left. (In other words, get in your ready position.)

3. All four connection points are used in the basics of the waltz.

4. The waltz basic (box step) consists of six counts (step, side, together, step, side, together).

5. The basics are more important than any other step. Make sure you know them and that you're comfortable with them before moving on.

6. The distinctive rise and fall gives the waltz an elegant look. Rise gradually happens on the second and fifth count; the fall occurs on the third and sixth count, and then gradually works its way into counts 1 and 4 as there's a slight lowering of the body.

7. Left turns (turning boxes) start on count 1 with the leader stepping front-left with his left. The conclusion of each three steps is approximately a quarter turn to the left.

8. Progressive basics consist of a series of fourth foot position steps in which both partners move simultaneously around the perimeter of the dance floor in a counterclockwise motion.

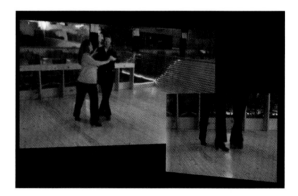

Next Steps

When you're comfortable with the waltz steps that you've gone through, you might want to look into learning more about leading, following, additional moves and patterns, or just more on the basics. Many different social groups exist for the sole purpose of dancing the waltz, and they can easily be found on the Internet by doing a search for your local area. The waltz is a very versatile dance because it can be done in the most formal settings, such as a wedding, or in very informal settings, such as in a park square. Enjoy dancing the waltz, and you'll add new dimensions to any social event you attend.

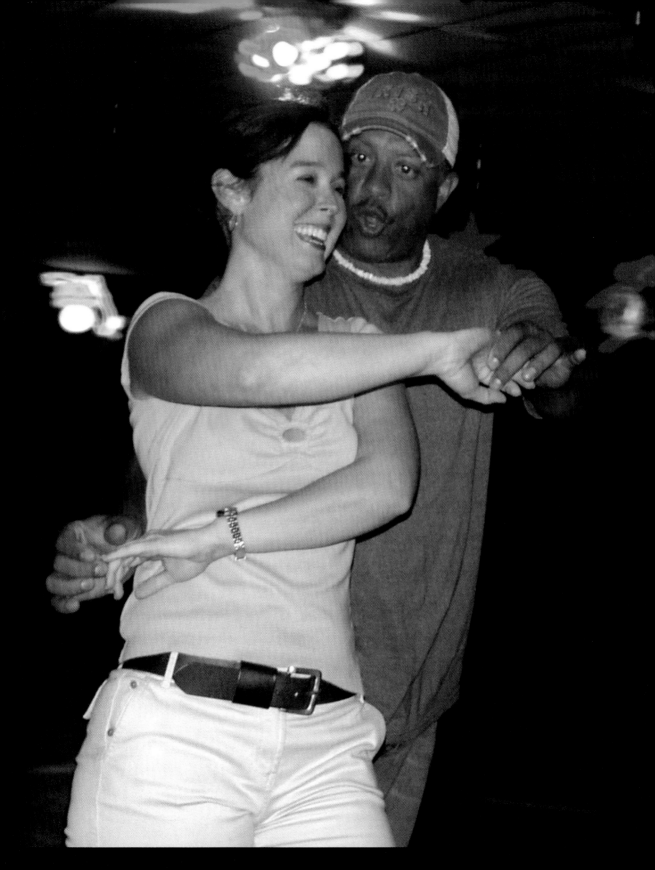

5

Picture Yourself *Two-Stepping*

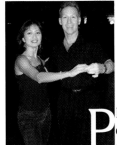

PICTURE YOURSELF navigating the crowded dance floor at a country-western nightclub. The acceleration in the two-step pattern is exhilarating as you execute the complex turns and spins that are trademarks of a great two-step. If you are the follower, the lights and the faces of your fellow dancers blur, with the exception of your partner's face, as you maintain a central focal point for the turns, pivots, and spins as the dance progresses around the floor. For the leader, it is a slightly different story. Your view of the dance floor is much closer to that of a video game; with each step your perspective changes as you advance around the floor, with new obstacles to avoid and your path constantly adjusting to the rapid changes on the dance floor. The leader's mind is rapidly clicking through the different moves available to him and fitting the best one to the immediate situation, ever mindful of the constant tempo of the two-step and his partner's placement. As you and your partner master this dance, the realization strikes that for the dancer, the two-step transcends the music—it is an exhilarating challenge in navigation and lead-and-follow dancing that is difficult to match in the genre of social dance.

The Six Ws of Two-Step

A STAPLE AT every honky-tonk bar with anything that resembles a dance floor, two-step (or Texas two-step) is arguably the most popular country-western couples dance.

Who Popularized the Two-Step?

The origins of the two-step are murky at best, but the two-step of today was popularized by fans of country-western music. However, the root dances were transported out West with the covered wagons during the nineteenth century with the emigrants who populated the Great Plains and beyond.

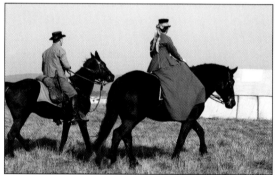

©istockphoto.com/Raymond Truelove

What Is the Two-Step?

The two-step is a smooth progressive dance created for four-quarter and two-quarter time music. It has a six-count basic that is counted quick-quick-slow-slow or one-two-three (four)...five (six). The time is the same as in the fox trot; however, the contemporary two-step does not use the box step as the fox trot does. Also, each step progresses forward around the dance floor, unlike in the waltz and the fox trot. The constant forward progression creates

an illusion of acceleration rather than a pause in a dance such as the waltz. The music that the two-step matches has a steady, even tempo with about 160 to 200 beats per minute. If you were to clap along, you would find yourself clapping evenly on every beat (one-two-three-four, and so on), unlike the waltz, where you would clap heavily on the first beat and lightly on the second and third beats.

> A *progressive dance* is one in which the partners dance around the perimeter of the dance floor in a counterclockwise direction. All of the turns, spins, and other moves are done while the partners are progressing around the floor.

The two-step is occasionally referred to as the *Texas two-step*; however, it is done throughout the country-western world.

Where Did the Two-Step Originate and Where Is It Typically Done?

Most histories agree that the deep roots of the two-step are the same as the waltz, with the predecessors of the two-step being the folk dances performed in the Bavarian and Austrian Alps. It appears that the waltz was adapted in the United States to match four-quarter time and half-time music. These dances grew into the fox trot and the two-step, with the two-step arising from the country-western subculture.

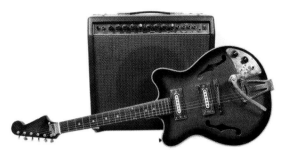

©istockphoto.com/kkgas

As a uniquely country-western dance, the two-step is typically done at a country nightclub. You will see two-steppers at any venue with anything close to a dance floor where country music is played. If you happened across a barn dance, you would most likely see line dance and two-step. You can also find a version of two-step in various ballrooms around the country, but it is not a staple dance in the ballroom circuit. Often, you'll find the two-step as part of a themed program for a country night or performance at a ballroom.

When Did the Two-Step Become Popular and When Is the Right Time to Two-Step?

The exact birth date of the two-step is unknown because two-step-like modified versions of the waltz have been danced since the mid-nineteenth century. That being said, the two-step as it is danced today emerged in the 1980s as a part of the resurgence of the country-western subculture. The dance of today is a highly evolved dance, with drastic departures from the lurching promenade of the 1970s.

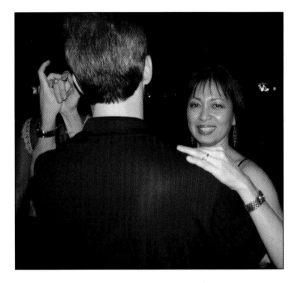

The right time to two-step is usually when the dee-jay calls the dance. In most country-western night-clubs, the deejay will announce what dance is appropriate for the song that is being played, as well as whether the song is designated for couples dancers or line dancers. It is an important rule of floor etiquette to pay attention to these indications. If you are not at a venue where a deejay announces the dances for each set or song, your ear is your best guide. You are listening for a song with between 160 and 200 beats per minute, in which the backbeat is very smooth and even. Because the two-step is danced to fairly quick-tempo songs, it is usually played early in the evening or early in each set of music.

Why Is the Two-Step Danced?

The two-step is danced to match a wide variety of country-western music. As far as partner social dances go, the two-step falls toward the less inti-mate end of the spectrum. It does not typically

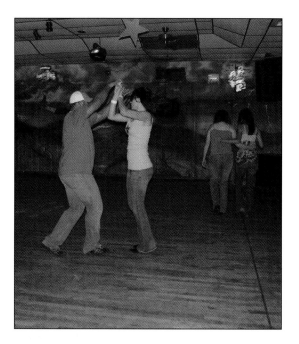

strong frame and rapid pace, it is a dance during which you could easily make an introduction to someone new and continue the conversation off the dance floor following the dance.

What Kind of Attire Should Be Worn?

Because the two-step is a country-western dance, country-western apparel or at least casual apparel is completely appropriate. If you own them, cowboy boots are appropriate for both men and women, whether you are in formal country or country-western black tie. For occasions when you are going out to a country-western nightclub, jeans are appropriate for both parties; however, if the woman wants to wear a casual skirt, that is also perfectly acceptable. There is and most likely always will be a part of American culture that dresses the country part to a T, with flouncy skirts for the women and western-cut plaid button-down shirts for the gentlemen, but in most parts of the country the majority of two-steppers have a mainstream look, with casual denim and nice shirts.

have the passion of the tango or the intimacy of a slow dance. It is a dance in which it is perfectly acceptable to dance either with a complete stranger or with a spouse of 50 years. With the

Visualize the Two-Step

BEFORE STARTING the lesson plan for each dance, it's recommended you take a few minutes to watch the DVD that comes with this book and view the current section. In this case, you'll be watching the two-step segment to allow your mind's eye to start processing ideas on how to get your body to do what you're watching. Visualizing the two-step will give you a good feel for what you're about to learn and will make the transition into reality that much easier.

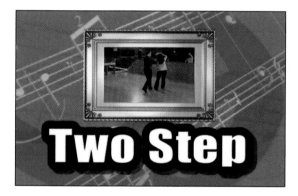

It's best if you watch the two-step section one time through without trying to do any of it. Just give your mind a chance to absorb the material so it's somewhat familiar to you when you hit replay to start the section over again. Watch how the dancers move around the dance floor (this one's not in place, so take note), think about the words that are used, and picture yourself dancing the two-step.

The second time you watch it, it's recommended that you take notes. Jot down the important parts of the two-step so you can engage other parts of the kinesthetic learning prior to getting up and dancing along. Write down what the connection

points are, what the basic steps are called, how many counts are in a basic, how to align with your partner, and so on. Also, write down any questions that you might have about the two-step. There's a good chance you will find the answer later on in this chapter, and if it's something you're already pondering, you'll be sure to remember the answer.

You'll find that by time you get ready to stand up and try the two-step with the DVD, the dancing won't be nearly as overwhelming. Writing down the key concepts will allow you to get a jumpstart on the rest of this chapter. You'll find that after you get up and try it, you'll probably have more questions. As this chapter goes on, the steps will be broken out with screenshots from the DVD, pointers will be given on where you should be during different parts of the dance, and frequently asked questions will be addressed that should satisfy most, if not all, of your questions and then some.

The third time you view the DVD, go ahead and dance along with it. See how far you can make it just by watching and trying. You'll probably find that one of the two of you is able to pick up and understand the material quicker than the other.

> **Just remember, everyone learns at a different pace. Be cognizant of this as you're learning with your partner. One of you might pick up certain aspects of the dance quicker than the other, and that's okay. Try to be patient and wait for the other person to grasp the material, and then move on.**

Now take a look at the rest of these pictures. All of them are taken of couples dancing the two-step. Some are more formal than others, but they're all doing the same steps. See whether you can visualize yourself dancing the two-step (the dance you just watched over and over) in all these different settings. Then, picture yourself doing the two-step at upcoming events or at local venues where you and your partner can go. Where will you go out dancing after you learn the two-step? Start thinking of the possibilities.

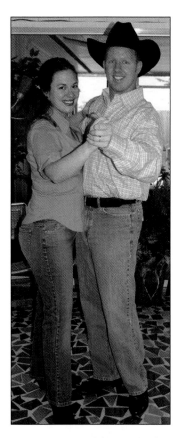

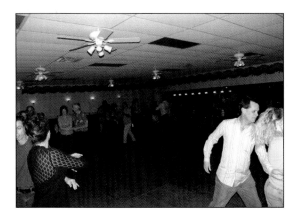

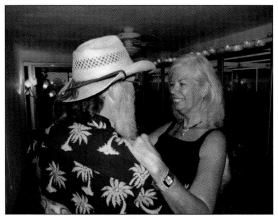

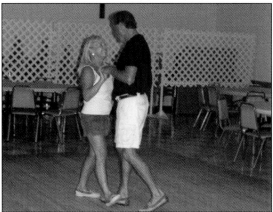

Two-Step Basics

THE TWO-STEP, by the nature of its background, is considered to be pure country; however, its roots show that it's more of a stretched-out descendent of the fox trot. Although two-step was once considered only a country dance, it has continued to grow into one of the most popular social dances around due to its leading and following characteristics and its eye-catching illusionary movements around the dance floor. Two-step is a smooth dance that offers much more than simply walking around the dance floor and dancing a pattern or two.

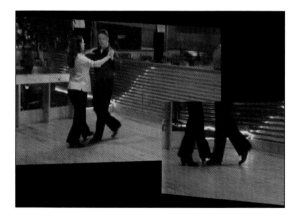

Several types of two-step exist, including Texas two-step, rhythm two-step, nightclub two-step, disco two-step, double two-step, and triple two-step. The two-step you'll learn here is the same as the Texas two-step and refers to the quick-quick, slow, slow rhythm in a progressive manner.

As previously mentioned, the two-step is danced to 2/4 timing, which means there are a great number of songs to practice to, including many from your favorite country music CDs or MP3s. As always, it might be best to do a search online for "two-step music," "two step music," or "2 step music" to stay current on what's playing now. At the very least, try to understand and get familiar with the timing in order to recognize the dance when the opportunity arises.

For two-step, the same two important rules apply that you'll continue to see throughout the book:

1. Ladies are always right! Ladies, put your weight on your left foot so you can be ready to start with your right. (This is what's called your *ready position.*)

2. Guys always get what's left. Guys, put your weight on your right foot so you can be ready to start with your left. (This is what's called your *ready position.*)

The Two-Step Basic

The two-step basic is composed of (are you ready for this?) two different timings, four total steps, and six counts of music. One more time on that one: two timings, four steps, and six counts. That's right! It's not as bad as it seems, though, because it's all done in a progressive manner and it's much like walking. Walking quickly and then slowly, then quickly and then slowly, then quickly...well, you get the point. The two-step basic, in layman's terms, is said out loud like this:

Quick-quick, slow, slow

If you're more mathematically inclined and like to use numbers, it's counted like this:

**One, two, three, five
(the four and six are held/silent)**

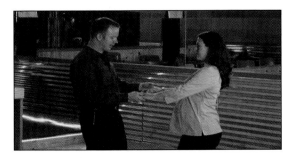

What Are Quicks and Slows?

Up to this point in the book, you've not used much more than walking-steps and touch-steps. The walking-steps that you went through in the waltz will be the most help in this chapter because they're used throughout two-step, just not with the same rise and fall as in the waltz. In two-step, you'll use almost all walking-steps (fourth foot position either forward or backward), but you'll do it in two different speeds, quick and slow, or as some people say, fast and slow.

In the two-step basic, there are two different speeds, quick and slow. *Quicks* take up one beat apiece and *slows* take up two beats apiece. The basic is said, "quick-quick, slow, slow," where the quick-quick is the first two beats (one each) and the slow, slow takes up two beats apiece, which ends up being counts 3 and 4 for the first slow and 5 and 6 for the second slow. For each slow, you take the step on the first beat and then hold the second one. (In other words, you don't step during the second beat of a slow.)

To summarize, following are some fun facts you should know:

▶ **The two-step is composed of two quicks and two slows.**

▶ **Each quick takes up only one beat.**

▶ **Each slow takes up two beats.**

▶ **A two-step basic takes up a total of six counts.**

It's also important to know that the speed of the step (quick or slow) should *not* determine its length. In other words, don't take tiny steps on the quicks because they're fast and then large steps on the slows. Your steps in two-step should be smooth and transparent to the casual eye so you don't look like you're going fast and then slow, then fast and then slow, and so on. The different speeds are best camouflaged by a steady and constant flow around the dance floor in a counterclockwise manner.

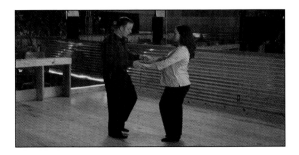

To try the two-step basics in place, assume foot position 1 and be in your respective ready positions. Next, you'll want to simply take a total of four steps in place, starting with quick-quick, then doing slow, slow. Remember, the quick-quick is 1-2, the first slow is 3-4, then the second slow is 5-6. Make sure to change weight each time and count the steps aloud (quick-quick, slow, slow, quick-quick, slow, slow or 1-2, 3, 5, 1-2, 3, 5, and so on).

Doing the basics several times in place should get you familiar with the timing and the changing of weight.

At the end of every six counts, you should be back in your ready position and you should be ready to step right back down on count 1 to start your quicks again.

> It's recommended you practice the quicks and slows for at least five to 10 minutes before trying them progressively.

Mirroring

When you're comfortable with the basics in place, go ahead and move into the next steps, which will allow you to do the basics of two-step without having to worry about anything but the footwork. To learn your individual steps the first time, stand directly in front of each other. Try facing each other, about two to five feet away from your partner in a mirrored position. It's important in two-step to see the opposite steps because both parties will need to understand what their partner is doing.

1. (Step 1 - Count 1) From a ready position, leaders will step straight forward with their left foot (fourth foot position), and followers

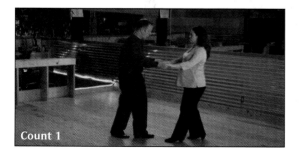

Count 1

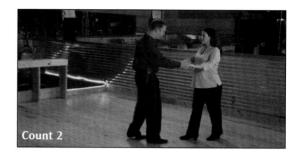

Count 2

will step straight back with their right foot (also a fourth foot position), with each partner changing weight to the foot that was moving by the end of step or count 1.

2. (Step 2 - Count 2) Leaders will now step straight forward with their right foot (still in fourth foot position), and followers will step straight back with their left foot (also still in fourth foot position), with each partner changing weight to the foot that was moving by the end of step or count 2.

> Because this is the first truly progressive dance you've learned here, it's important to mention the passing of the knees and feet, or what's called *keeping your legs together*. When you step continuously either forward or backward in fourth foot position, your knees should nearly brush each other as they pass during the transition from one step to the next. Don't take stutter-steps, and avoid having your knees more than one to two inches apart if at all possible. It's particularly unattractive, for obvious reasons, to watch either partner move around the floor with his or her legs wide open.

3. (Step 3 - Counts 3 and 4) Leaders will again step straight forward with their left foot (still in fourth foot position), and followers will again step straight back with their right foot (still in fourth foot position), with each partner changing weight to the foot that was moving by the end of count 3 and then holding count 4. (In other words, no stepping during count 4.)

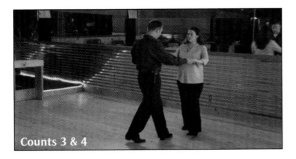

Counts 3 & 4

4. (Step 4 - Counts 5 and 6) Leaders will now step straight forward with their right foot (still in fourth foot position), and followers will step straight back with their left foot (also still in fourth foot position), with each partner changing weight to the foot that was moving by count 5 and then holding count 6, (In other words, no stepping during count 6.)

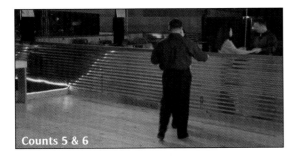

Counts 5 & 6

Now that you're able to do a complete basic down the line of dance (did we mention that it's counter-clockwise yet, and that the men are typically going forward and the ladies are going backward?), go ahead and practice what you just learned with music over and over or just continue trying it without music. If you'd like, you can both go forward down the line of dance or you can both go backward as well, just for practice purposes and to get the timing.

This is the part where it'd be best to do several miles of two-step (no joke) before you ever try to put it all together while dancing it for the first time. Trust us on this one. Try going for walks and saying and trying your quicks and slows or even trying them when you're shopping or just walking around the house. Leaders, you might want to count out loud to give the follower a chance to match you step for step each time you start. This means the leaders would say, "Ready, and," or "5-6-7-8," or "Ready, go," or whatever they're most comfortable with, and then step with their left foot.

> **If either partner gets on the "wrong foot" during the exercise, just stop, laugh, and start up again after the leader counts it off . . . 5-6-7-8, and you're back dancing again.**

Practice doing the two-step until you're both comfortable with the steps and the answers to each of the following questions:

▶ **Should my feet come together or pass while I'm doing quicks?**

▶ **How many steps do I take during the six-count basic?**

▶ **What foot position am I always in if I'm walking forward or going backward?**

▶ **Which part of the slow do I step on, the first part or second part? Which one is held?**

The Two-Step Basic as a Couple

Now that you're both experts on doing the basics as you walk down your street or at your favorite grocery store, it's time to try them together as a couple. Are you sure you're ready and that your feet can do the quick-quick, slow, slow once your upper body is engaged? Well, if you skipped right to the dancing and didn't practice it on your own, you might have a tough time figuring out where any problems are if they arise. Practicing before coming together is critical to building the confidence of each partner, and it's easier if you come in with steps that are closer to being set in stone with your body. Again, ballroom or social dancing is not all skill; in fact, it's probably closer to only about 25-percent skill, with the remainder being your attitude. If you're excited and ready to practice and learn, chances are you'll zip right through any problems that you encounter and you'll be all set for a great time.

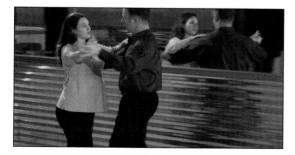

Your toolkit for the two-step basic includes:

▶ **Foot position 1 (ready position to start and at any time during the dance when you have to start over)**

▶ **Foot position 4 (all forward and backward steps of the basics)**

▶ **Connection points 1–4 (all will be used in the basics)**

▶ **Six-count basic (remember: a total of four steps in the basic)**

Are you ready to start two-stepping with your partner? Here goes. First, you'll want to get into your closed dance position with your partner (use all four connection points) and be in your ready position. Also, you'll want to make sure you're slightly offset so no one gets stepped on. Leaders, go ahead and give your countdown (5-6-7-8 or however you choose) and move forward by stepping with your left and then with your right (quick-quick), then slow it down a bit and do your first slow (two counts), and then do your second one. Now, start it over again and do all four of the steps back to back to back to back—quick-quick, slow, slow—and now, just repeat it over and over. Fantastic, you're doing the two-step! Keep going and see how far you can make it. Go slow, though—this isn't the time to try to run over your partner.

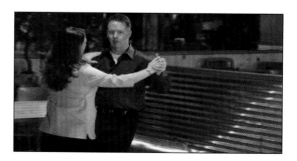

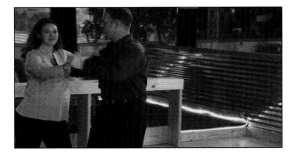

As usual, it's now time to make sure this is true lead-and-follow dancing. Get back to your ready position and let's make sure the leaders are actually leading this one and the followers are following it. Leaders, just like in any dance, you have four connection points that you'll use here to help you out. The two most important ones for the leaders are connection points 1 and 4, while the follower must focus on connection points 2 and 4. Although neither the leader nor the follower uses connection point 3, the elbow, as a primary indicator, it is important for both parties to maintain this connection point. Connection point 3 supports the connection between connection points 2 and 4. Leaders, your upper body must be in synch with your lower body on this one because you'll need to drive toward your partner as if she wasn't there. Your arms should not be pushing; rather, your upper torso will guide her along with a constant forward pressure, just as though you were walking at her without using your arms. Consider your arms mere extensions of your body, with the connections simply there for her to feel your body moving toward her.

Did it work? If so, you did each of the following (you should aim for at least three of the four):

> ▶ **You successfully completed the six-count basic (all four steps).**
> ▶ **You both changed weight four times during the basic.**

> ▶ **You managed to keep her directly in front of you (slightly offset).**
> ▶ **You kept a smile on her face or caused one.**

To recap this one, the leads that take place in the two-step basic are fairly straightforward (no pun intended). The follower should be able to feel the leader coming directly toward her with connection points 1 and 4, which should tip her off as to the fact that she should be stepping backward and out of the way. The leader's forward momentum should leave no doubt as to the direction or speed that both partners should be traveling. Each step of the basic here should pass the other, and both partners should only end up in the ready position when there's a stopping point, such as when someone gets on the wrong foot and you start over during the dance. Otherwise, the traveling momentum will allow both partners' feet to continue moving down the line of dance, and the feet should not come together. Success, as usual, is marked when everything is working together and both partners are moving effortlessly with one another and not stepping on each other's toes.

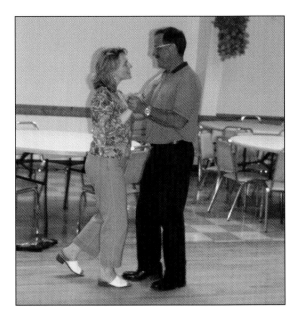

For the Followers

Followers, this next part is the same as it is in any dance: If the leader isn't perfectly clear on the lead (in other words, the motion or the guidance), don't move! This is especially true in the two-step because everything happens so quickly that there's not much time to react. Now, of course, you shouldn't be stubborn and just stand there, but if the lead isn't nearly perfect as he steps toward you with confidence, make him improve it. Focus on the problem if there is one. There shouldn't be much of an argument here—either you feel it and it's enough or you don't. The only major thing you need to concentrate on here is being in good frame so you can feel connection point 4 and sitting slightly back into connection point 2.

For the Leaders

Leaders, we continue to emphasize the following point: If you give a lady a choice (on the dance floor), she'll take it! If you leave the door open for interpretation, you never know what you'll end up with. Okay leaders, take your partner in closed dance position slightly offset (all four connection points) and try the basics again. Practice the basics from a starting point over and over until you're comfortable with starting directly into the quick, quick. Then, have your follower close her eyes and see whether she can follow what you're doing and when you're starting. It helps if you lean slightly forward to start the motion prior to the first quick. This will allow your partner's body to start moving, which will cause the step. If the lead is right, your partner will match you with step for step and also in speed. If the follower is having difficulty (other than not understanding the basics), there's a better than 90-percent chance it has something to do with the lead.

Turning on Corners

The ability to dance in a straight line as you move down the line of dance (counterclockwise) is one thing, but at some point you'll encounter your first corner (if you haven't already). When you get there, don't panic. Corners should be treated in the same manner in which you'd take one if you were driving (and driving sober, mind you). Corners should be taken with ease, nice and rounded where possible (not so much that you turn the square or rectangular dance floor into one big circle, though).

For the Leaders

As simple as it sounds, taking your partner from going straight backward to a 90-degree turn can be quite challenging. It's during this part that many followers get stepped on and the frame for both partners gets broken. It's up to the leaders here to make this work, so take note. As you're nearing a corner or the end of any given straightaway, you must start preparing your partner for the turn. This happens by gradually stepping a little more left (somewhere between forward and front-left) and by lifting your right elbow ever so slightly to offset the follower's weight. It doesn't matter whether it's on the quicks or slows, just that it starts happening. Lifting slightly with your right elbow, or connection point 3, will shift the follower's weight from a position of being balanced to one that sends her weight to the back-right (the direction you're turning). You'll want to keep your partner directly in front of you (still offset, but in front of you) as you take this turn, and make sure you maintain all four connection points. It should end up being as simple as you walking forward and then rounding a corner without question. The follower should never even know what is going on. The figures on the next page show a visual depiction of your steps.

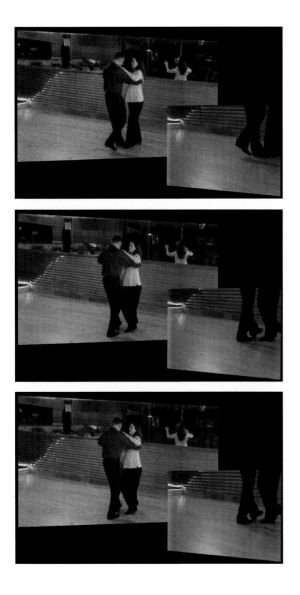

give you the right signals; otherwise, there's a much greater chance of you running into someone else, getting stepped on, or, worse yet, getting accused of back-leading on the dance floor. The right signals for you should be a slight turn of your body to the right, a slight lifting of your left elbow (which will cause your weight to head in a back-right motion), and the visual interpretation of what your partner is leading. Don't try to step anywhere other than straight back from your hip. If your body is turned, you'll be stepping in the correct direction. Leave it up to the leaders to put you in the right position for it.

Stopping on the Dance Floor

This next part might seem a bit too elementary, but rest assured it will turn out to be one of the most useful bits of two-step knowledge that you'll get. The ability to stop moving down the line of dance in an instant is critical! It's the equivalent of having a new set of brakes on your car. While dancing the two-step around the perimeter of the dance floor, many, many different things can happen, and the leader is typically the one who has to see and react to what's going on. From the occasional spilled drink on the floor, to someone walking out in front of you, to a fast-turning line dancer who happens to lose control, there are many different reasons why it's imperative to understand how to stop. Information for both leaders and followers is coming up.

For the Followers

Followers, we'll make this one simple for you. You'll just worry about doing your steps backward and then staying with your partner. You'll be stepping straight back until you near the corner, then you'll be stepping somewhere between back and back-right. Now, don't start turning on your own. It's imperative that you wait for your partner to

For the Leaders

Leaders, your right hand (connection point 2) has 85 percent of the responsibility when it comes to stopping your partner. Ten percent of the responsibility comes from your body's ability to stop, and the other five percent is given to your left hand to help balance out the equation. You should practice dancing and stopping on a dime (a figure of speech). Truly, though, leaders, see whether you can do a couple of basics, then stop your partner's momentum just by stopping her with your right hand (almost as if you were trying to catch her in your hand). Although the momentum stops, the basics shouldn't, and both partners should revert to doing the basics in place until forward or backward momentum once again resides. Leaders, just be prepared at any point to stop your partner in her tracks and change direction or speed to keep the dance going. Leaders, it's also your responsibility to keep others from running into your partner. If someone or another couple is heading directly for your partner, do not hesitate to remove your hands from connection point 1 or 2 to stop the other person with an open hand (not a fist or anything that would cause pain). Just politely stop the other person before your partner gets hit, stepped on, run into, or anything else out there on the dance floor.

For the Followers

Followers, you also get a chance to apply what you've learned here. There will be times when you'll see something happening on the dance floor that the leader doesn't, and you'll want to ensure that he either stops or that you stop whatever is going on prior to it impacting your partner. For example, there will be times when you'll be going forward down the line of dance rather than backward, and you'll see someone stopped in front of you. Simply take your hand out of connection point 2 and quickly place it over your partner's right shoulder to stop his momentum. Go on, give it a try. The leader should be moving backward until you stop his weight, and then you'll both be doing your steps in place until he either changes directions or starts moving again.

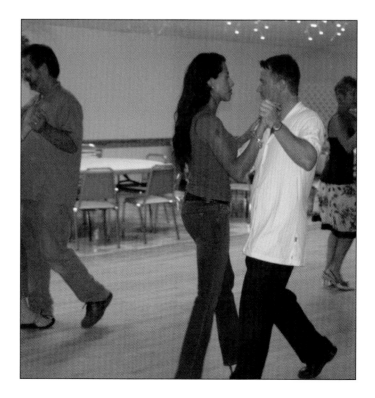

Fun Drills to Put It All Together

FOLLOWING ARE a number of drills and exercises set up specifically for you to practice what you've learned. Instead of just picturing yourself doing the two-step, this is where you'll put it all together and dance it all for yourself. Try to go through each one of the drills because they focus on different elements, leads, and thinking patterns. By the end of these drills, you should feel confident enough to try out your two-step almost anywhere.

Drill 1: The Chair Dance

This is one that you can do right where you're sitting, or while you're at work or at the dinner table, or heck, almost anywhere. You'll focus on the steps and the timing of each one. As you sit, you'll first put your feet in the ready position, then you'll start taking very small, discreet steps in place while you count to yourself, quick-quick, slow, slow . . . quick-quick, slow, slow. What you're doing here is starting to get the rhythm into your head while you're putting your feet in action. It's a good idea to practice a few minutes here and a few minutes there, but not for long sessions because you'll wear yourself out while you're sitting. This is a fun exercise that is best done alone or in a discreet manner unless those around you have a vested interest in your dance success.

Drill 2: Going the Distance

Three kilometers, five kilometers, or 10 kilometers—how far you go depends on when you're comfortable with the basics of two-step. You can do this exercise alone, with your partner, or with a group. Set up in your ready position and start walking on the quicks, then do your slows. Quick-quick, slow, slow . . . quick-quick, slow, slow—over and over and over until it becomes so ingrained into your muscle memory that you do it without

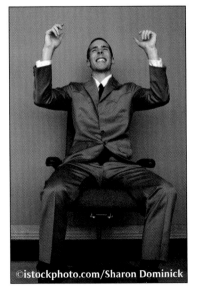
©istockphoto.com/Sharon Dominick

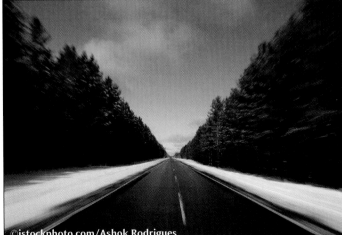
©istockphoto.com/Ashok Rodrigues

thinking. Practice the steps going forward, backward, around corners, in place, and around any obstacles that turn up. You can even set up as though you're in frame to practice, which will help you feel like you're dancing. (Beware, the number of odd looks goes up dramatically if you're doing this on the side of the road.) Count your steps out loud so that you hear them as well.

Drill 3: Slow, Medium, and Fast (Three Different Speeds)

Set up in your ready position, but this time with your partner, and test several different speeds of the two-step. You don't need music to do this, just a leader who's willing to try it at his own pace, literally. When the leader is going very slowly, you'll see that it takes quite a bit more control than when the dance is faster, and the ones in the middle will feel very comfortable. If you have two-step music, go ahead and give some songs a try.

Drill 4: Red Light, Green Light

Here, leaders, you'll work on the starting and stopping of your progressive two-step. The intent of this drill is to deliberately force both the leaders and followers to get a handle on the momentum changes that are frequent in two-step. Leaders, what you'll do here is set up with your partner and start dancing around the perimeter of the dance floor or whatever room you have to practice in. Then, on frequent occasions, you'll practice stopping your partner's momentum and then starting right back up again. Pretend you continuously have someone stepping out in front of you and you keep having to hit your brakes. The basic footwork won't change during this exercise because you'll continue with the basics as you stop and start over and over.

Drill 5: Driver's Ed

This is a fun exercise to do with groups of people as well as with just a single couple. Around the perimeter of whatever dance space you're practicing on, you'll want to set up a number of obstacles to navigate around. Set them up in a manner that would force the leader to constantly move his partner in different directions to avoid hitting them. The obstacles could include such household items as chairs, laundry baskets, garbage cans, fake trees or plants, or just about anything else that could be visible, yet not so obtrusive that neither partner can get by. After the obstacles are all set up, the leaders get to practice the basics in and out of all the obstacles. The exercise reinforces and demands control from the leader and forces the leader to continuously think ahead while looking over his partner's right shoulder.

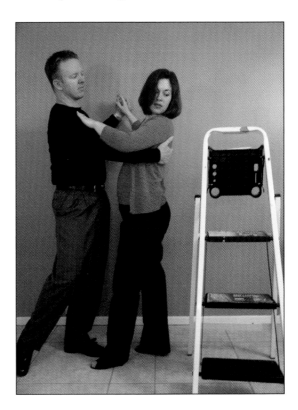

Hot Tips for the Two-Step

A S ONE OF THE best-recognized country-western dances around, you should now have a good feel for what the two-step is all about. Following are a number of tips and pointers that have been put together for you to go through to help reinforce what you've learned.

▶ Two-step is a fast-moving dance that requires both partners to keep their heads up and their eyes open. Either partner looking down detracts from the look of the dance, throws off the balance of the couple, and could easily cause accidents on the dance floor due to the dancer not paying attention.

▶ Two-step should be smooth, almost like gliding. Dancers should look as though they're effortlessly moving around the floor. Up and down (vertical) motion should not be visible as the couples execute the basics.

▶ The size of the steps taken in two-step should be determined by the follower's gait. In other words, if the follower has long legs, the leader will have to stretch a bit to make her feel comfortable; conversely, if the follower has a short stride, the leader has to adjust and dance to the step size of his partner.

▶ Maintaining frame and connection is critical in the two-step. The leader must be able to move in any direction at all times, and all connection points must be engaged for effective maneuverability.

▶ Offset your feet to start the dance. Leaders, your right foot should be between the follower's two feet because your first step is toward your partner. If the leader is directly in front of his partner, and his partner doesn't move, someone's getting stepped on. Don't start your dance this way! Also, having your feet offset enables both partners to be able to look over the shoulder of the person they're dancing with.

▶ Be aware of your surroundings and others on the floor.

▶ The basics in two-step are terribly important. Spend more time practicing the quick-quick, slow, slow than anything else. When you have it down, it'll be easy to add moves. If you try to do moves too quickly, you'll set yourself up for a long, hard road.

▶ The continuous flow of movement should be prevalent in the two-step. If it looks or even feels like it's choppy, it probably is. The fluidity seen in the two-step is a result of using natural body movements rather than stiff-legged patterns.

▶ Pass your feet! This enables you to avoid the look of skipping, hopping, or stutter-stepping around the dance floor.

Review and Next Steps for Your Two-Step

G REAT JOB! If you're starting from the beginning, you've now completed three dances. To ensure that you're comfortable and to do a final recap, we'll run back through the major points of what you've learned. Go through each one and come back to this list as necessary for a quick review.

Review

1. Ladies are always right! Ladies, put your weight on your left foot so you can be ready to start with your right. (In other words, get in your ready position.)

2. Guys always get what's left. Guys, put your weight on your right foot so you can be ready to start with your left. (In other words, get in your ready position.)

3. All four connection points are used in the basics of the two-step. Connections 1 and 2 are the most important for the guys and 1, 2, and 4 are the most critical for the ladies.

4. The two-step basic consists of six counts: quick (1), quick (1), slow (2), slow (2).

5. The basics are more important than any other step. Make sure you know them and that you're comfortable before moving on.

6. The smooth glide of the two-step is distinctive and is enabled by the passing of the feet in a continuous motion around the perimeter of the dance floor. Don't close your feet in the basics.

7. Left turns (turning when at a corner) start with the leader stepping front-left with his left. Typically it's done on the first quick, but it can also be started on the first slow. Regardless, the corners are typically taken in a gradual, rounded movement.

8. Stopping two-step momentum is critical in avoiding accidents. The leaders have the responsibility of watching their surroundings and reacting if necessary. The majority of the lead is done with connection point 2.

Next Steps

When you're comfortable with the two-step basics, you might want to look into learning more about leading, following, or additional moves and patterns. A quick Internet search will likely reveal several places in your hometown where the two-step is danced. The two-step is a fairly versatile dance that can be done in a ballroom, but it's most typically found in country nightclubs or at local dance events. Have fun dancing the two-step. The aerobic exercise alone from the miles of two-step will get your endorphins in gear while you add pleasure to your next outing.

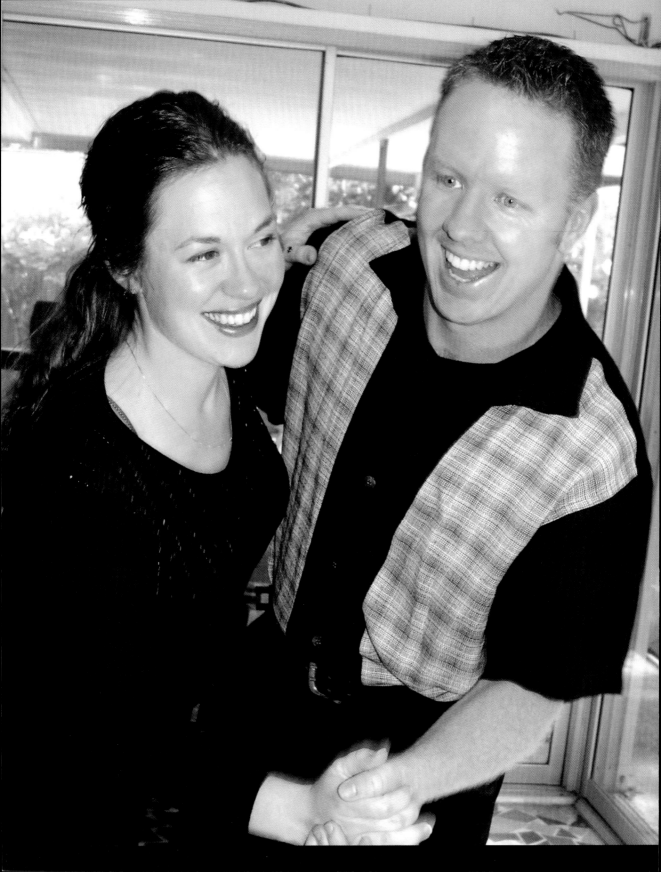

6

Picture Yourself

Swing

Dancing

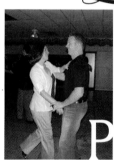

PICTURE YOURSELF in two-tone shoes bopping to the upbeat music popularized during the Big Band era and beyond. You and your partner are enjoying the fast tempo, manageable footwork, and innumerable dance moves offered by swing. As you dance, you settle into the strong, elastic connection characteristic of swing, with the relaxed handhold and frequent movement toward and away from your dance partner. The relatively stationary nature of the dance allows you to practice on any size dance floor or, for that matter, almost any size corner of a crowded dance floor! As you practice your new skills, you are finding yourself dancing swing at more and more venues—you couldn't have done without it at that class reunion, and at your coworker's wedding last week you and your partner were the talk of the table. Swing dancing enabled you to get out there and heat up the dance floor more frequently than you ever thought possible. You are now swing dancing at specific swing events in your area, as well as at local nightclubs and almost every dinner and dancing special occasion that has come up. The timeless swing will not go out of style any time soon with its toe-tapping beat and snappy dance moves.

The Six Ws of Swing

ONE OF THE MOST popular dances of the twentieth century, swing can be seen at almost any event where there is couples dancing. The exuberant music and look of swing attracts dancers of all ages and all walks of life.

Who Created and Popularized Swing?

Swing was created by the African-American community in Harlem to match the jazz and swing music of the day. It was popularized by such swing icons as Herbert White, who formed Whitey's Lindy Hoppers, and by dancers such as Frankie Manning and Dean Collins, who firmly planted swing on the big screen. The filmmakers of the 1930s took the Charleston, Lindy hop, and swing from Harlem and included clips in the newsreels of the day as well as

a few key movies, but it was Dean Collins who truly made a place for swing on the silver screen by teaching it to top contemporary Hollywood dancers whose performances were then included in more than 100 movies between 1941 and 1960. Swing was further modified and homogenized for the masses by Arthur Murray and his national chain of ballroom dance studios.

What Is Swing?

Swing describes a family of dances that were born to express the strong beat of jazz, blues, big band, and bop music. The forefathers of the modern East coast swing that you are learning in this chapter are the Charleston and the Lindy hop. From these eight-count dances the jitterbug was born in the 1930s with a six-count basic. Swing as you are learning it in this text has a six-count basic that is described as slow, slow, quick-quick; one (two), three (four), five-six; or side, step, rock-step. Swing is a spot dance, but don't let that fool you—you'll be doing a whole lot of moving around to the hopping beat!

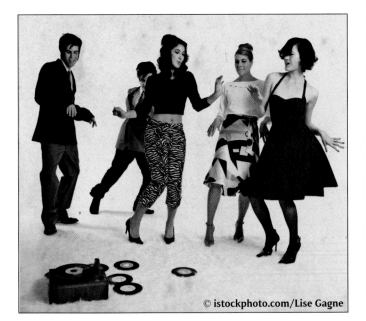
© istockphoto.com/Lise Gagne

A *spot dance* describes any dance in which the partners dance for the most part in one spot on the floor. Also called a *stationary dance*, a spot dance basically centers around a central point, with the partners turning, changing directions, and rotating around that point.

Although swing is a spot dance, there is a lot of motion created, as previously mentioned. This motion can be primarily described as vertical, like a bouncy ball. The swing is a rhythm dance (the opposite of smooth), with expansive freedom of expression and interpretation in connection points and style.

Where Did Swing Originate and Where Is It Typically Done?

As previously mentioned, swing was born in the nightclubs of Harlem in New York City, largely on the dance floor of the illustrious Savoy Ballroom.

Swing has found a home at almost any event with dancing, with the exception of events where the music and dancing is exclusively Latin. You can learn a version of swing at your local ballroom, and you will most likely see swing dance in many forms at wedding receptions or class reunions. You can also dance swing at a country-western nightclub! However, for the true swing enthusiast, a swing dance is the ultimate place to tap your toes. Chances are, if you turn to the Internet or just start asking around, you won't have to look long to find your own local swing-dance club. These sub-communities dance at various local venues are occasionally tied to a dance studio, but are populated by enthusiasts from all walks of life.

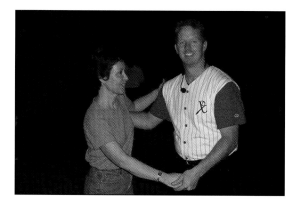

When Did Swing Become Popular and When Is the Right Time to Swing?

The Charleston and Lindy were born in the 1920s, with the six-count jitterbug following in the mid-1930s. As previously mentioned, swing gained an immense amount of exposure on the silver screen starting in the late 1930s. Swing received another boost from the soldiers, sailors, and officers of the United States Armed Forces as they took the swing dance from base to base and from base to hometown during the 1940s. From there, the ballrooms caught onto the craze led by the Arthur Murray studios; however, at this point the ballrooms took the opportunity to distill swing down to the bare essentials to make dance a possibility for the less-than-nimble-footed public. From there, swing became a permanent part of our culture.

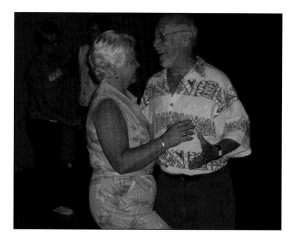

Swing dance is appropriate anytime a song with the correct tempo and beat combination is played. It is an upbeat dance with very strong aerobic attributes. So, you must also be prepared for a great workout if you want to swing dance. Also, in the interest of your own safety and the safety of those around you, make sure you have enough space. Although swing is much more controlled than its predecessors, the Charleston and the Lindy hop, you still run a risk of getting kicked or stepped on if you are on an overcrowded dance floor in an exuberant crowd.

Why Is Swing Danced?

Swing is danced as a physical manifestation of the energetic music by which it was inspired. For many, it is danced as a celebration of youth, as a return to their own youth, or as a representation of the energy and vivacity the dance requires in its full glory.

What Kind of Attire Should Be Worn?

There is no dress code or standard apparel for swing, so the rule of thumb is to dress appropriately for the venue you are attending. If you do choose to become involved in a local swing-dance club or group, you will probably immediately notice that a number of members or participants put a great deal of effort into vintage period dress, down to the zoot suits for the men and bobby socks and full-skirted dresses for the ladies. For many people this is almost as important to their experience as the dance itself.

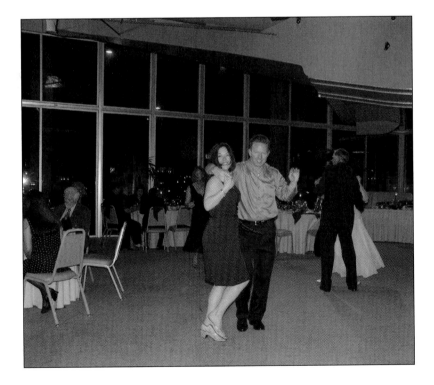

Visualize the Swing

BEFORE STARTING the lesson plan for each dance, it's recommended you take a few minutes to watch the DVD that accompanies this book and view the current section. In this case, you'll be watching the swing segment to allow your mind's eye to start processing ideas on how to get your body to do what you're watching. Visualizing the swing will give you a good feel for what you're about to learn and will make the transition into reality that much easier.

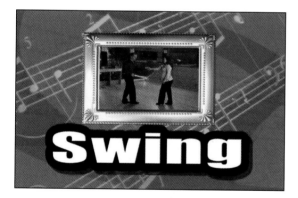

It's best if you watch the swing section one time through without trying to do any of it. Just give your mind a chance to absorb the material so it's somewhat familiar to you when you hit replay to start the section over again. Watch how the dancers move, think about the words that are used, and picture yourself dancing the swing.

The second time you watch the DVD, it's recommended that you take notes. Jot down the important parts of the swing so you can engage other parts of the kinesthetic learning prior to getting up and dancing along. Write down what the connection points are, what the basic steps are called,

how many counts are in a basic, how to align with your partner, and so on. Also, write down any questions that you might have about the swing. There's a good chance you will find the answer later in this chapter, and if it's something you're already pondering, you'll be sure to remember the answer.

You'll find that by time you get ready to stand up and try the swing with the DVD, the dancing won't be nearly as overwhelming. Writing down the key concepts will allow you to get a jumpstart on the rest of this chapter. You'll find that after you get up and try it, you'll probably have more questions. As this chapter goes on, the steps will be broken out with screenshots from the DVD, pointers will be given on where you should be during different parts of the dance, and frequently asked questions will be addressed that should satisfy most, if not all, of your questions and then some.

The third time you view the DVD, go ahead and dance along with it. See how far you can make it just by watching and trying. You'll probably find that one of the two of you is able to pick up and understand the material more quickly than the other.

> **Just remember, everyone learns at a different pace. Be cognizant of this as you're learning with your partner. One of you might pick up certain aspects of swing quicker than the other, and that's okay. Try to be patient and wait for the other person to grasp the material, and then move on.**

Now take a look at the rest of these pictures. All of them are taken of couples dancing the swing. Some are formal, some are very informal, but they're all doing the same steps. See whether you can visualize yourself dancing swing (the dance you just watched over and over) in all these different settings.

Then, picture yourself dancing swing at upcoming events or at local venues where you and your partner can go. Where will you go out dancing after you learn the swing? Again, there are many possibilities, so start thinking of them.

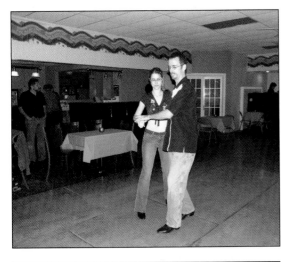

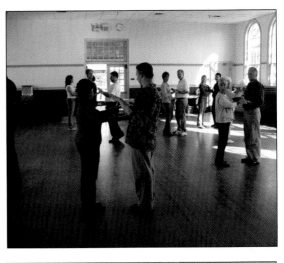

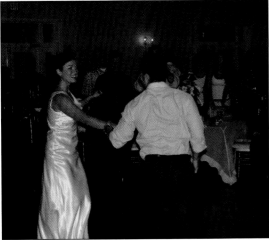

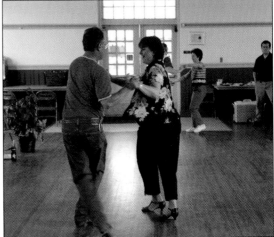

Swing Basics

SWING DANCING is best known for its fun up and down motion (lilt) and elastic tendencies. There are three main variations of the swing basic, which include single rhythm, double rhythm, and triple rhythm. All three of them are part of the standard six-count basic, and they can be done interchangeably throughout the dance. You'll first learn the single rhythm and then get exposed to the double and triple as the chapter progresses. You'll also learn when they can be used best.

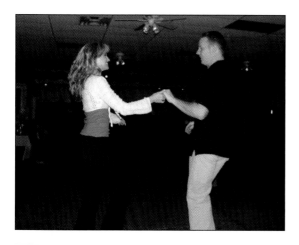

Single rhythm **equates to taking one step for every two beats of music (later described as a** *slow***).** *Double rhythm* **equates to taking two steps or having two foot motions (in other words, a step and a touch) for every two beats of music (the equivalent of a** *quick-quick***).** *Triple rhythm* **equates to taking three steps for every two beats of music (later described as a** *triple-step***).**

The swing is danced to either 2/4 timing or 4/4 timing, which means the number of songs to which you can practice is quite extensive, whether you're just turning on your radio or pulling out your CD or MP3 collection. For specific songs or up-to-date playlists, it might be best to do a search online for "swing music" and find a few songs from whatever genre of music is your favorite, and then practice along. You should familiarize yourself with the swing beat and with the timing in order to recognize the dance when the opportunity arises. Before you begin the swing, let's recap the two most important rules:

1. Ladies are always right! Ladies, put your weight on your left foot so you can be ready to start with your right. (This is what's called your *ready position.*)

2. Guys always get what's left. Guys, put your weight on your right foot so you can be ready to start with your left. (This is what's called your *ready position.*)

The Six-Count Basic

The six-count basic of swing is made up of two slow steps and two quick steps. It starts out with a slow to the side (which means you step on count 1 and then hold count 2). The second step replaces the weight onto the foot that is now free without much movement (in other words, your free foot came off the ground and then right back down in the same spot) on count 3 (another slow, which means count 4 is held with no stepping). The last two counts are done with rock-steps in which each partner rocks back on count 5 and then replaces his or her weight on count 6, ready to step into a slow to start the basics over again.

> The quick-quick, slow, slow or slow, slow, quick-quick (the same thing, just with a different starting point) can be found in the basics of two-step, hustle, swing, and fox trot. It's good to know that after you get the rhythm down, you'll have the basic timing set for several different dances.

Swing, in layman's terms, is said out loud like this:

Side, step, rock-step,

Side, step, rock-step

If you're more mathematically inclined and like to use numbers for your steps, it's counted like this:

One, three, five, six,

One, three, five, six

For the look and feel of the correct lilt, you'll want to let your shoulder and body lower slightly on the first slow in the direction of your step (this can be attained by flexing your knee), rise back up and square to your normal framed position on the second slow, and then keep your body fairly level for the rock-step to allow you to regain your composure and balance before starting again. This slight up-and-down motion will give you the feeling that you're matching the up-and-down heartbeat of the swing song that is playing, which will allow you to get into the character a little easier. If you're feeling flat-footed or stiff-kneed, now is the time to work on it. Think of it as putting a little bounce in your step or a little bop to the music. You'll want to play around with it until you're comfortable or until your partner says it looks good once you learn your steps.

To try the swing basics in place (you can stand next to one another for this one), assume foot position

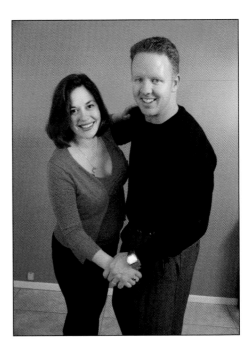

1 and be in your respective ready positions. Next, you'll want to simply step down on count 1 (changing weight), then step down on count 3 (again, changing weight), then step quickly on steps 5 and 6 (also with changes of weight). There are a total of four steps taken over six counts. Try them with the counts now, and it'll sound like this: 1 – 3 – 5-6, 1 – 3 – 5-6.

Now try the same pattern with the rock-steps, where count 5 is now done in either a third foot position or a fifth foot position (rather than straight back), where you're now taking two steps in place (slow, slow on counts 1 and 3), then doing the rock-step on 5 and 6. You have slow, slow, rock-step, or step, step, rock-step. Doing this a few times should get you familiar with the timing and the changing of weight. At the end of every six counts, you should be ready to start back over on count 1 with your first slow. And, just in case you were wondering, you will *not* end up in your ready position at the end of each basic, so keep that in mind.

Mirroring

When you're comfortable with the basics, go ahead and move into the next steps, which will allow you to do the basics of swing without having to worry about anything but the footwork. To learn your individual steps the first time, stand directly in front of each other. Try facing each other, but be about two to five feet away from your partner in a mirrored position. It often helps if you're able to see the opposite steps, if for no other reason than just to validate your own.

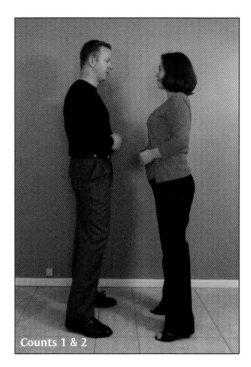

Counts 1 & 2

1. (Step 1 - Counts 1 and 2) From a ready position, leaders will step off to the left with their left foot (second foot position) and followers will step off to their right with their right foot (also to the second foot position), with each partner changing weight to the foot that was moving by the end of step or count 1. Count 2 is held with no foot movements because it's part of the slow.

2. (Step 2 - Counts 3 and 4) Leaders, step with your right foot to the right about shoulder-width apart from your left foot (second foot position). Followers, step with your left to the left about shoulder-width apart from your right foot (second foot position). Although it says to step to the side, your free foot here should just have to step down from where it was and, if done properly, it will end up in the second foot position. Again, make sure to change weight to the free foot on count 3 and then hold count 4 because it's part of the second slow.

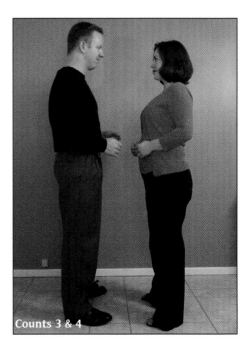

Counts 3 & 4

3. (Step 3 - Count 5) Leaders, step with your left foot to the back-right into a fifth foot position. Followers, step with your right foot to the back-left as you step into a fifth foot position as well. Make sure you change weight to the foot that was just moving because this is the first part of your rock-step. This step is where many errors occur in swing due to dancers not changing weight. Rock onto this foot and then be ready to step again on the very next count.

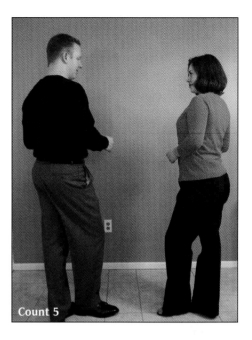

Count 5

4. (Step 4 - Count 6) Leaders, you'll now change weight back onto your right foot because it will be in front of your left. Changing from count 5 to 6 here will give you the rocking motion because your left foot is in back and your right foot is in front. Followers, you'll change your weight onto your left foot because it'll be in front of your right foot. Changing from count 5 to 6 for you will be the same because it will give you the rocking motion from back to front. Each of you will still be in fifth foot position at the end of count 6, and you should now be ready to start back over with step 1 and count 1.

Be sure to keep your rock-step under control. If either the leader or the follower takes too large of a step back in the rock-step, it will throw you off beat.

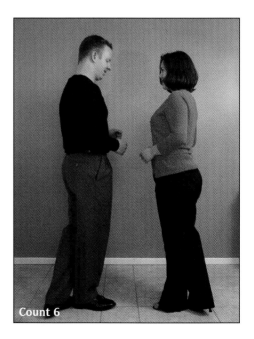

Count 6

When you're both able to do a complete basic, then another, then another, go ahead and practice what you just learned with music. It'll be the last thing you try before putting it all together. Leaders, count out loud to give the follower a chance to match you step for step when you start. The leader should say "Ready, go" or "Ready, and" on the counts 5 and 7 (the equivalent of slow, slow) just prior to starting. The 5 and 7 here refer to the music that you're listening to as you prepare to take your first step. Think of the old dance movies in which they give a countdown of "5-6-7-8" before starting. This is the same thing, but because you'll be starting with slows, it's best to start on that timing. To start, it'd be like this: "Ready, and" slow, slow, rock-step. This should make it easier for both partners.

Practice until you're both comfortable with the steps and the answers to each of the following questions:

> ▶ At the end of each basic, should you be in your ready position or in fifth foot position?

> ▶ Are there any steps that you'll take in a six-count basic that do not include a change of weight?

> ▶ How many steps are taken in the six-count basic?

> ▶ What are the foot positions typically used for steps 1 and 3, and 5 and 6, respectively?

As always, if either partner gets on the "wrong foot" during the exercise, just stop, laugh, and start up again after the leader counts it off. . ."Ready, and," and you're back dancing again.

The Six-Count Basic as a Couple

You should now be an expert on doing the basics by yourself. As such, it's now time to try them with your partner and see what happens. If you've practiced the basics enough on your own, you'll be able to focus on just the new material that's about to be introduced. Leaders, this is especially important for you because you don't want to be learning to lead at the same time as you're learning your steps. If you skipped right to this section and didn't practice it on your own, you might have a tough time figuring out where any problems are if they arise. Practicing before coming together is a critical building block; the confidence each partner brings makes it much easier because you'll both have high expectations. As repeated in many places in this book, social dancing is probably close to 25-percent skill and 75-percent attitude, so keep up the excellent work and positive reinforcement.

Your toolkit for the swing basics includes:

> ▶ Foot position 1 (ready position—to start only)

> ▶ Foot position 2 (counts 1 and 3 of the basic)

> ▶ Foot position 5 (counts 5 and 6 of the basic)

> ▶ Connection points 1–4 (all will be used here in the basic)

> ▶ Six-count basic (essential for the swing to work)

Okay, get into position and start your swing. The first thing you want to do is get into your dance position with your partner (use all four connection points), have your feet offset, and be in your ready position. Wait, before you go any further.... Leaders, take your left hand and go from the normal connection point 1 level to one that is down closer to the waistline. Next, instead of having your hand cupped, you'll want to take your left palm and place it across the top of the follower's right hand and close your fingers around the side of it, so your four fingers are now touching her palm (see the pictures below). The reason for this is to make it a little less formal and a little more comfortable to add to the swing feel. Also, having connection point 1 lower makes it easier to dip down slightly with the lilt that you've been working on. Okay, leaders, go ahead and give your starting count of "Ready, and," and step to the side with your left and then to your right with your right, then bring your left back and do the rock-step. Now that you got through one basic, just repeat it over and over. Okay, you're doing the basics now . . . side, step, rock-step, or slow, slow, quick-quick . . . . Fantastic!

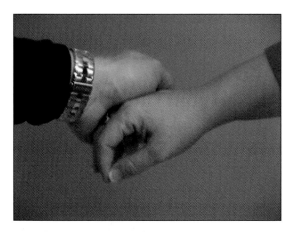

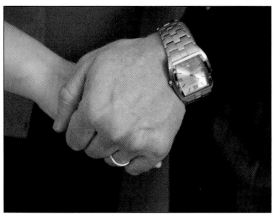

Now that you've done it a few times and you're feeling good, let's dissect the lead-and-follow portion of the dance to ensure that both of you understand what is happening and how it's all broken down. Leaders, we'll focus on your part and work through what we need for success. All four connection points will help you out on the swing basics. The three most important ones for you to start the swing are connection points 1, 2, and 4. Leaders, you've got a lot to put together here to make sure everything is in synch (upper body and lower body), so we'll break it down for you to make it as clear as possible.

For the Leaders (Mostly)

Leaders, to give your partner a clear, unambiguous lead, you'll first need take your left hand (connection point 1) and move the follower's hand to your left (her right) to get her weight moving in that direction. When you bring it to the side, you'll also bring it down a couple of inches, which will cause her right shoulder to dip. (Remember the lilt.) At the same time, you'll raise your right elbow (connection point 3) a couple of inches, which raises her left shoulder and tilts her body to her right. The final piece is done with connection point 2, where the leader's right hand (the palm of it) will move laterally to the left and guide the follower so she cannot stay over her left foot (essentially sending her to her right foot). The complex part here is that all three of these things happen simultaneously during the first step. The easy part is that they all make perfect sense when you think about what has to happen to change the weight of an object to put it into motion. (Sorry, ladies, that was for analogous purposes only.)

Leaders, for the second step (counts 3 and 4), you'll need to bring your partner back to your right so she can put her weight on her left foot prior to the rock-step. To do this, the exact opposite of everything you did on the first count must occur. Your right elbow (connection point 3) will drop slightly as it moves back to the right, your left hand (connection point 1) will come back up at a diagonal to the right as it provides a nice, easy pushing sensation to the follower's right hand, and your right hand (the fingers part) will pull slightly off to your right to help put the follower onto her left foot. Wow! Easy, right? Maybe. You might want to try to isolate each of these movements to make sure they're working in parallel. Start from the preceding paragraph and work through this one. The whole thing takes about three seconds, so be prepared for a lot to happen at once. It might not all work together the first time or the second, but as long as you both understand the concepts, you should be in good shape.

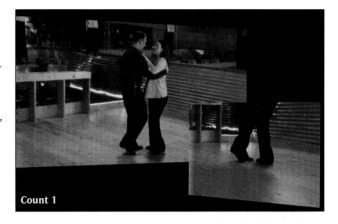

Count 1

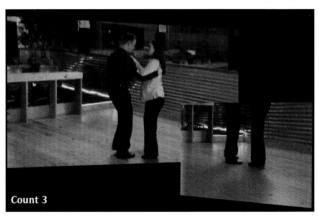

Count 3

Okay, the rock-step. It only took a few times to get the step on your own, so how hard can it be? Well, let's see if we can sum it up by giving another analogy for both of you to try (just so you both understand what's happening here). Do your rock-steps on your own for a minute in a pretend dance position (in other words, not touching). When you rock back, think of yourself sword-fighting and at the exact time that you're doing the "rock" part of the rock-step, use your connection point 1 hand to thrust the sword at your opponent, who's directly across from you. This means your hand will be thrusting away from your body while your body is moving backward. Go on, try it. Not as easy as it seems, is it? This motion should simulate what the leader has to do in that he'll be rocking back and also pressing his left hand forward to cause the follower's right hand and frame to go backward, which causes the follower's right foot to rock back.

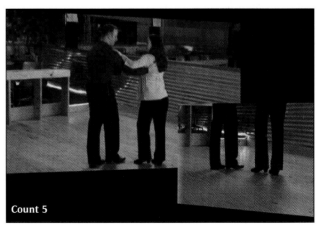

Count 5

So, leaders, let's see whether we can apply it here—not with a "thrust," but rather a nice, easy push away as you rock back. With your right hand (connection point 2), you'll also be letting the follower move slightly away from you and you'll let the finger part (as opposed to the palm or the entire hand) open up a little more in order to let the follower's right shoulder and right foot move backward for the rock-step. On count 6 (the "step" part of the rock-step), the leader's sole goal should be to place the follower onto her left foot while getting himself onto his right foot to be ready to start again. The easiest way for this to happen is for the leader to shift the follower's weight forward on that final step (remember, the follower just rocked back on her right foot, and her left foot should be in front) by using connection points 1 and 2 together at the same time.

Now, finally, try to put it all together with all that thinking stuff—and make it look and feel natural! Sure, the basics seem easy enough on their own, but if you really want to dance lead-and-follow swing, understanding the physics behind each and every move is a must. It will apply to every move that you'll learn from here on out. Guys, the more you understand about how to "manipulate" the woman's body, the better off you'll be. Ladies, the more you know about what feels right and why, the better you'll be at following because you'll know how to compensate when needed and you'll know when to just sit back and enjoy the dance.

Go ahead and dance through the swing basics a few times. Did it work? If so, you did or felt each of the following (you should aim for at least five of the six):

► You successfully completed all six counts.

► You both felt completely overwhelmed with all the details of the lead.

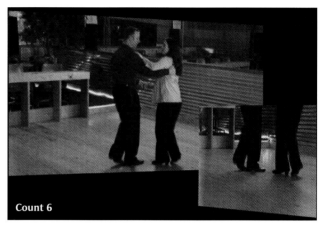

Count 6

► You managed to stay directly in front of one another.

► You felt a bit uncoordinated, yet more intelligent for understanding.

► You both had a smile on your face or caused one with your perplexed look.

► You weren't satisfied with the basic, but you were optimistic because you're getting better.

To recap on this one, there are several different leads going on during the swing basic. The follower should feel as though her body is completely in the hands of the leader. There should be enough going on that the follower could literally do the steps blindfolded. On the first step, the leader essentially tips the follower's body and gets her to step to her right. On the second, he shifts her weight and sends her back onto her left foot. Then, on the third step (count 5), he sends her away from him as he steps back, and then he brings her back together with him on count 6 for the fourth and final step. You put all that together in a well-executed slow, slow, quick-quick or side, step, rock-step, and you're all set. It's as simple as that! Once it works, you'll want to practice it over and over again until you're completely comfortable.

Though more time is spent here, it's essential because you'll apply these concepts in almost every swing move you'll learn. If there's a part you don't understand, you might want to contact a local professional to get it worked out. Success is marked when everything is working together and both partners are moving effortlessly with one another.

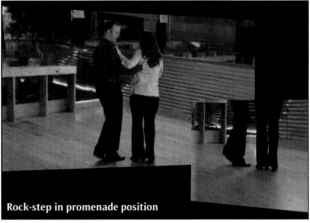

Rock-step in promenade position

Right Turns

Remember back when you did the right and left turns in the slow dance? If so, the next two sections will be a breeze. The leads are almost identical (the only distinction being that swing has the lilt), and you'll just have to incorporate the basic rhythm of the swing. The step-by-step guide is broken out for leaders and followers separately, but you should both try to learn the footwork for both partners to give you a better perspective of what's happening with your partner. Start with doing one basic, then stop and get ready for your next one. (Remember, you're not in your ready position at the end of a swing basic.)

Leader's Footwork

Leaders, on the right turns, you'll make a change to your basic on the second slow only. The first slow will remain the same, just as it did in the slow dance, then on the second one, instead of changing weight back to your right foot without moving, you'll step off a quarter turn to your right (or slightly less if you're more comfortable). When you step, though, you're not going to step "forward and right"; you're just turning your foot (pretty much in place, except for a new direction) and stepping back down onto it. Once you're firmly on your right foot and facing a new direction, you'll bring your left foot up and do the normal rock-step behind the right. (In other words, you're not going to leave your left foot facing the original direction.) So, what you have here is the following: side, turn, rock-step, side, turn, rock-step. Before you get too

much further, make sure you practice just this part until you have it. Each time you start, you should be facing a new direction somewhere off to your right (a quarter turn, or some derivative thereof—more or less will depend on the lead that accompanies the step, which you'll read about soon enough). Below is the visual depiction of the two slows.

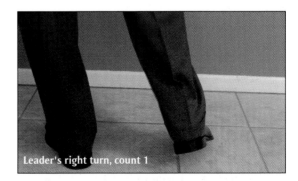

Leader's right turn, count 1

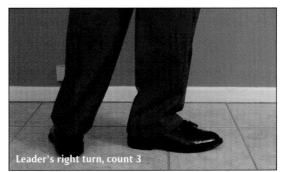

Leader's right turn, count 3

Follower's Footwork

Followers, you guessed it: Your steps are the exact opposite on this one. There's no change to your first slow, but on the second, you'll step forward and slightly to the right with your left foot, while doing a quarter turn to your right. Ladies, if you think about stepping directly in front of your right foot while you're turning your body, it should make it easier for you. Once you've turned on the second slow, all you've got to do from here is your rock-step, so bring your right foot up to your left, put it in fifth foot position, and go for it. Practice these turns until you're comfortable, and then try them together with your partner. Just remember, at this point you're now a different direction from where you started (off to your right as well). Below is the visual depiction of your slows.

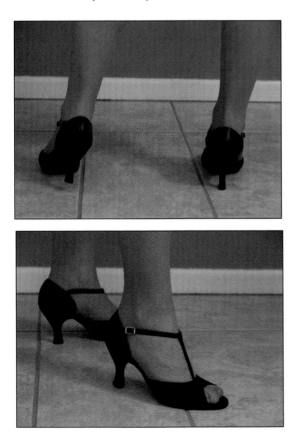

How the Right Turn Is Led

Luckily, you don't have to worry about your steps because you should know them pretty well by now. What you do have to understand is how right turns are led, so that's what you're about to see. Just like with the steps you just learned, there is no difference on the first slow. Good, one part down! While we're at it, there's no difference on the rock-step either. Excellent, two parts down! That leaves only the second slow (counts 3 and 4) to do anything on. Okay, leaders, what you've got to do here is place the follower in front of you (and slightly offset to your right) as you do a quarter turn to your right (just like the right turn in the slow dance). When you do so, you'll take your second slow with your right foot directly between her two feet. This means that you have to get her past you prior to stepping.

The majority of the lead here will come through connection point 2, and it will seem as though you're pulling her. In addition, though, there's also a steady rotational lead that will come from the leader's upper torso as everything moves together at once (including connection point 1, because it will be pushing slightly up and to the right to assist with the weight change). Leaders, once you have her there and balanced (if done correctly, you're now facing a new direction and your right foot is pointing directly between her two feet), you can go into the rock-step.

As soon as you get it once, go back and try again, then again, then again. Leaders, you can test your own lead here by doing more of a turn and less of a turn, just to see how it works and what is enough and what isn't. It's imperative that you know your limitations, so take this one out for a test drive. There are no specifics, so don't tell yourself that you're doing it wrong if you're not turning enough or too much; leave that to the follower because she'll be glad to tell you. Last point, followers: If it's comfortable and feels right, it probably is. Let the leaders know what you're feeling. If the lead is too strong or not strong enough, convey this as well and work on it together.

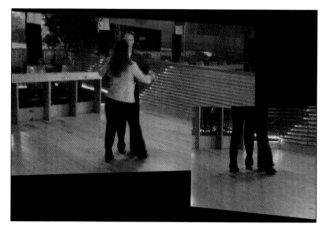

Left Turns

Now that you're able to do your basics and then do them with right turns, you've got to add in some left turns so you don't end up getting too dizzy to complete the dance. Following is the same break-down as we'll first go through the leader's footwork, then the follower's, then how to lead the move.

Leader's Footwork

Leaders, on the left turns, you'll make a change to your basic on the first slow only, as opposed to the second one as you did in the right turns. On the first slow, instead of stepping to the left as usual, you'll turn approximately a quarter turn to your left and step left at the same time. When you take your step, take it just a tad smaller than you normally would because the follower has a bit farther to step than normal. When you've completed your first slow, do the second one as you normally would (remember, you're in a new direction), and then there's no change to your rock-step. Each time you start, you should be facing a new direction off to your left (a quarter turn or some derivative thereof; more or less will depend on the lead that accompanies the step). At the right is the visual depiction of the two slows.

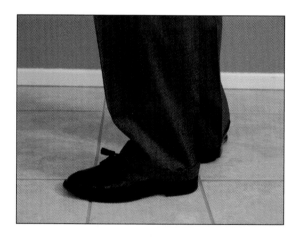

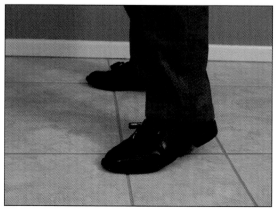

Follower's Footwork

Followers, as usual, your steps are the exact opposite on this one. The change here is to your first slow, then the rest of it's the same. On the first slow, you'll step forward and slightly off to the right while turning your body and aiming your right foot to the left (that was a mouthful). Go through that one slowly—it makes sense. When you've completed the first step, the second (your second slow) should be normal, with the only difference being you'll have to square your left foot up with your right prior to stepping in place. The rock-step is the same from your basic. Work through it a couple of times on your own, then put it together with your partner. At the right is the visual depiction of your slows.

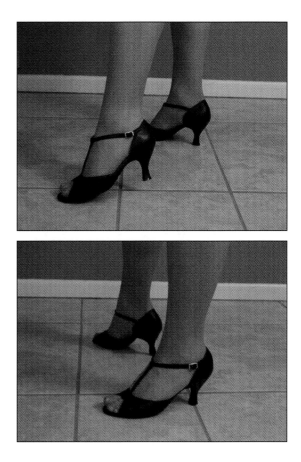

How the Left Turn Is Led

You're now getting a better feel for the leading and following. Guys, when you go to lead the left turn, everything has to work together again. (Maintain your frame.) Connection points 1 and 2 (fingers and palm) are most important. Leaders, as you step and turn to your left, you have to ensure that your upper body communicates the same thing to your partner. Connection point 1 will serve as the guide and must pull slightly to help with the direction change. Connection point 2 is used to ensure her shoulders are turned (use your fingers for this) and to help send her weight in the new direction (use your palm for this part). When you've completed the first slow, the leader reverts back to the basics to complete the remainder because the rest is the same. You can say it like this: Turn, step, rock-step, turn, step, rock-step. Practice, practice, practice, then move on to the next part.

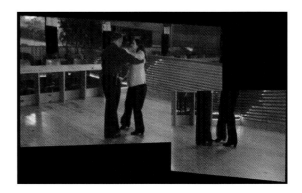

Underarm Turn (Outside Turn)

To give a little jump and jive to your swing, you'll now add in some fun underarm turns. Underarm turns are not as simple as the guys lifting their hands and the ladies starting to twirl, but they aren't terribly difficult either. The steps and leads will be broken down, and you should both be able to execute these turns within the next few minutes.

Leader's Footwork

Leaders, your footwork does not deviate much from the normal basic. The first change will be on the first slow. You will step front-left (somewhere between an eighth of a turn and a quarter turn) rather than straight out to the side. The second slow will remain the same as that in your basic. Next, your rock-step. Rather than stepping into the fifth foot position with your left foot, you'll rock back into the fourth foot position because you'll want to rock directly away from your partner, who'll now be in front of you (and also rocking away from you). Make sure the rock-step is small and in control. Upon completion, you can go back into the basics or you can do another underarm turn just for practice.

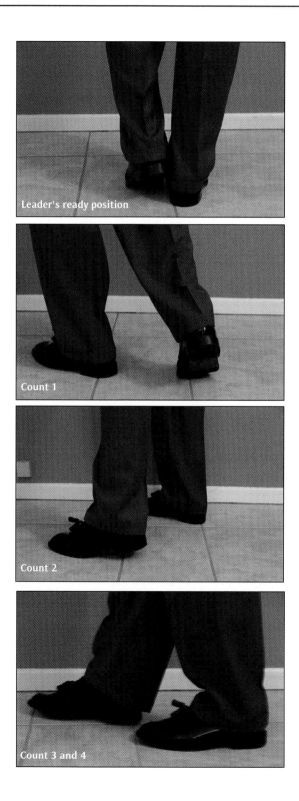

Leader's ready position

Count 1

Count 2

Count 3 and 4

Follower's Footwork

Followers, this is your first chance to really deviate from the normal side-to-side basics in the swing. What you won't deviate from is the slow, slow, quick-quick timing because it's imperative that it remains the same while you're turning. Okay, are you ready? On your first slow, you'll step out with your right foot and do a quarter turn. Your weight and center point should now be steadily over your right foot as your body is starting to turn. On the second slow, you'll continue your momentum in a forward direction while you do a half turn to your right to face your partner. You'll only take one step, and it'll be with your left foot at the end of the turn, but on your second slow.

At this point, you'll have done a total of three quarters of a turn off to your right with just two steps. (Replace the slow, slow with turn, turn). Notice it's not called a *spin*. You won't be spinning at all because that would suggest that you're out of control. You're doing one small turn followed by another that has a bit more momentum. After the second slow, you'll be ready to do your rock-step, but you'll do it straight back in a controlled fourth foot position. This is to allow you to catch your weight and send it back forward. Don't take a large step back, or else you'll end up really far away from your partner, and you'll both be thrown off. Make

sure the rock-step is small and in control. Upon completion, you can go back into the basics or you can do another one just for practice.

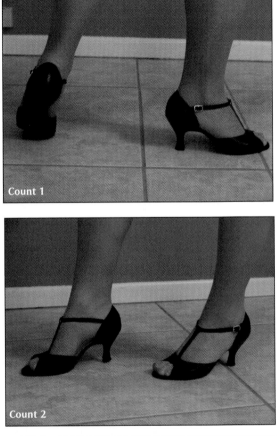
Count 1

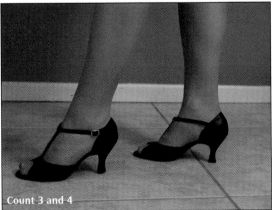
Count 3 and 4

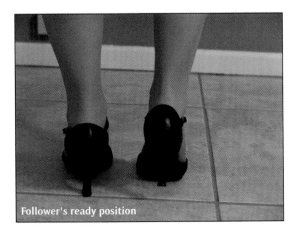
Follower's ready position

How the Underarm Turn Is Led

The best way to think about the lead here is like an overpass on a road and a vehicle passing through underneath. The overpass has to have a gradual slope (as opposed to straight up and down) that has enough clearance for the vehicle to pass underneath without knocking off the vehicle's roof. First things first, leaders, you have to give the followers advance notice of the turn. The notice is given on the first slow as your left hand goes from waist-level on top of her hand to a palm-to-palm connection slightly above the follower's shoulder, as if to block her from coming any closer to you (see the first picture below). At the same time, leaders, you'll bring the follower in a little closer to you to give you more weight (via pressure) to direct her momentum as you have to have her through the turn by the second slow. The clue here for the ladies is that your right hand has now shifted from

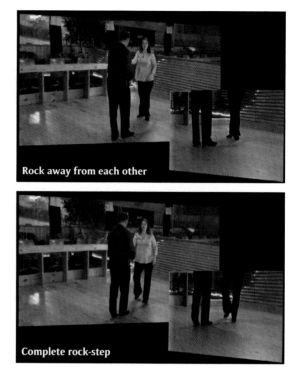

Rock away from each other

Complete rock-step

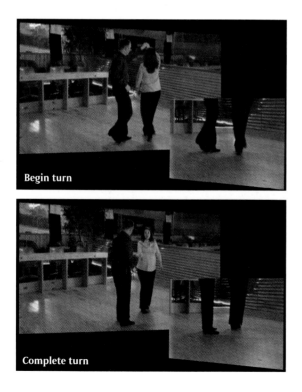

Begin turn

Complete turn

waist-level to above your shoulder, and you now feel as though your momentum is compressing into the leader's left hand.

At this point, leaders, you'll provide the on-ramp by raising your left hand (taking hers with you) as you move it off to the left at an upward diagonal. At the same time, you'll use your right hand (connection point 2) to send your partner under the overpass (a bridge could also work here). The sending of your partner through means you'll use your right hand and guide her (not push her abruptly) as far as you can before she slides out of your reach. Once she gets through the hole (overpass), you'll bring your hand down as though it were an off-ramp (not a cliff). Bringing the hand down and keeping it in the center of the two of you will help her unwind and square up with you by the second slow. This all happens quickly, but it all happens.

Once you both do the second slow, you'll rock away from each other and regain your composure for either another basic or any other turn that you might try. Often, an inside turn is followed by an underarm turn; however, that move is not covered in this text.

All right, how about a little checklist here for leading this one? We'll walk through it step by step to recap it for you.

▶ **Leader shifts connection point 1 from waist-level to just above shoulder-level by the first slow.**

▶ **Follower steps to right (up to a quarter turn) on the first slow as weight starts heading in that direction.**

▶ **Leader provides overpass for follower to quickly move under (complete with on-ramp and off-ramp) prior to stepping down on second slow.**

▶ **Connection is reestablished at second slow and partners have middle-point to regain composure and then to execute rock-step.**

▶ **Rock-step is done in fourth foot position to allow for backward momentum of followers.**

When you're able to do it over and over without problems, you'll be ready to put it all together with the next page full of fun drills. Enjoy while you learn!

Fun Drills to Put It All Together

WE'VE PUT TOGETHER a number of fun drills and exercises for you to go through to work on your swing. Instead of just picturing yourself doing the swing, you'll put it all together and dance it for yourself. Go through each of the drills as they focus on different moves, leads, and thinking patterns. Soon, you'll feel confident enough to try your swing dance anywhere.

Drill 1: Shadow Dancing

Set up in your ready position in your dance frame and do the basics on your own. Have your partner do his or hers as well, just not with you. Turn some music on and dance through everything you just went through, including the basics, the left turns, the right turns, and the underarm turn. See

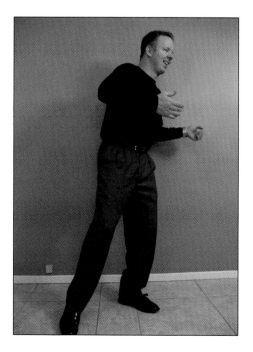

who can last the longest without messing up, stopping, or getting off beat. Basically, both of you will be swing dancing individually, running through the leads and/or follows and footwork for all of the moves in your repertoire to music to cement them in your memory.

Drill 2: The Turtle and the Hare

Set up in your ready position, but this time with your partner, and test several different speeds of the swing. No music is necessary, but it helps if you have it because you'll have fun practicing slow, normal speed (you'll decide what normal is), and then as fast as you can handle.

Drill 3: Open or Closed?

Here, you get to double the number of swing moves that you learned just by changing your position. Leaders, as you're dancing your basics, drop connection point 2, move slightly away from your partner, extend your hands to offer an open dance position, and keep the basics going. You still have to lead the basics, but now you'll do it with both of your hands in front of you. Same concepts, just different hand positions. After you master the basics again, try the left and right turns, and then the underarm turn. It can all be done! Then, mix and match and go from a closed dance position to an open dance position at random times while you practice the moves. It'll keep you both interested and entertained. For more of a challenge, leaders, try dropping your right hand as well and dancing only with your left hand (you still have to lead it). The basics are more exciting this way (one-handed), but the other moves might get a little tricky.

Drill 4: Look Ma, No Hands!

On this one, leaders, you'll go from a closed dance position to one in which you're leading only with your right hand (still in closed position). You'll drop connection point 1 and lead everything with the right side of your body (connection points 2, 3, and 4). The three connection points all still hold the frame as this, too, adds another cool look to your swing and makes for fun practicing.

Drill 5: Hula Dancing

Using a hula hoop is a great way to practice the leading and following for the swing. Leaders, you're in charge as usual, and followers, you just need to set up inside the hoop with your arms around the outside and your hands wrapped back up under and on the inside of the hoop itself. Practice everything you learned in this chapter. This can be done with or without music.

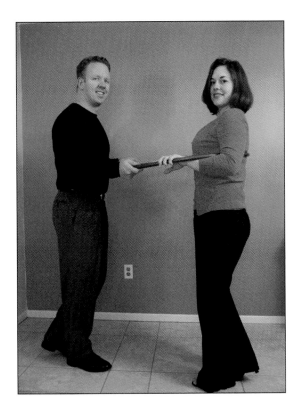

Hot Tips for the Swing

THERE'S TYPICALLY no doubt what makes for a great swing song, but there is when it comes to what makes for a great swing dance. Following are a number of tips, pointers, and reminders for dancing swing now that you know enough to be dangerous. Keep these in mind as you dance more and more and get out to practice.

▶ **Keep your steps fairly small, especially during the rock-step.**

▶ **Don't overextend your arms during the basics. This is the fastest way to pull someone else's arms out of their sockets. Stay close to your partner and in control, and you won't have any problems.**

▶ **Swing, by default, is fun! Having a good time on the dance floor is more important than being technically correct on everything but not enjoying it.**

▶ **Aerials might look great, but should never be done with an unsuspecting partner. Never attempt any kind of lift, drop, kick, or throw with a partner you've never danced with or practiced with. If you do choose to do any acrobatics, you and your partner should work with a professional, and you should always be very careful if you do them on the social dance floor. There is a good chance that you are putting other dancers on the floor in more danger of injury than yourself or your partner. Awareness of your surroundings is critical.**

▶ **The up-and-down motion (lilt) helps give the look and feel of a boppy swing if done correctly because it gives you a little bounce in your step. Too much motion detracts from the lead and can cause motion sickness and a lack of willing dance partners.**

▶ **Keep your head up. You don't have to look into your partner's eyes, but you should have your head up at all times and appear alert and interested. Having your head down gives the appearance that you're more interested in your feet than you are in your partner, and much of the dance is lost.**

▶ **The basic steps in swing are the most important. Do them well, and you'll be able to do almost anything out on the social dance floor. Practice them until they become second nature so you can dance with anyone.**

▶ **Enjoy the dance. Above all else, try to enjoy dancing the swing. Take in the surroundings, the music, the atmosphere, the feelings, and so on.**

Review and Next Steps for Your Swing

HOT DIGGITY DOG! You're doing great—another chapter down, and you're that much closer to an awe-inspiring look out on the dance floor. To ensure that you're comfortable and to do a final recap, we'll run back through the major points of what you've learned. Go through each one and come back to this list as necessary for a quick review. Start at the beginning and work your way through each point.

Review

1. Ladies are always right! Ladies, put your weight on your left foot so you can be ready to start with your right. (In other words, get in your ready position.)

2. Guys always get what's left. Guys, put your weight on your right foot so you can be ready to start with your left. (In other words, get in your ready position.)

3. All four connection points are used in the basics of the swing, but you can also do the basics with just connection point 1 (single-hand hold or two-hand hold), or just connection points 2, 3, and 4 (without 1).

4. The swing basic consists of six counts (slow, slow, rock-step) and is more important than any other step because it's the one you'll be repeating over and over and over.

5. Left turns start on the first slow, and right turns start on the second slow.

6. Rock-steps are done in fifth foot position for the basics (which gives them a more open look), but they are done in fourth foot position after moves such as the underarm turn,

when the partners are separated yet facing one another.

7. Underarm turns are to include early clues for the follower to assist with the lead. Clues include the shifting of hand positions, the changing of momentum, and a slight, yet even pressure on the body to move in a particular direction.

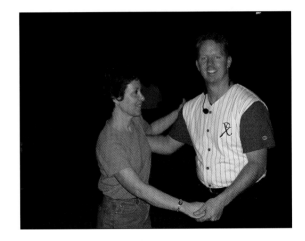

Next Steps

As soon as you've mastered all the footwork and cool swing stylings, you'll want to get out and go learn some more. Whether it's more about leading, following, additional moves and patterns, or just the basics, there are plenty of places to learn. There is typically no shortage of swing dance groups, and they can easily be found on the Internet by doing a search for your local area. Swing is, has been, and always will be a very popular dance that can be done in almost every setting. Get your dance shoes back on, and get out there and join the fun.

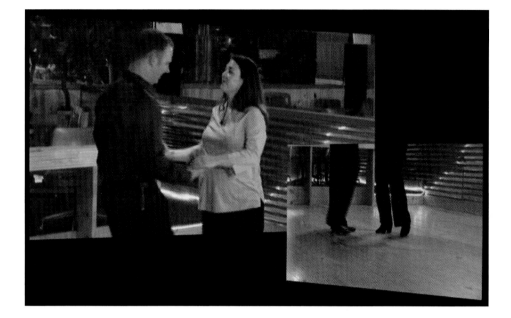

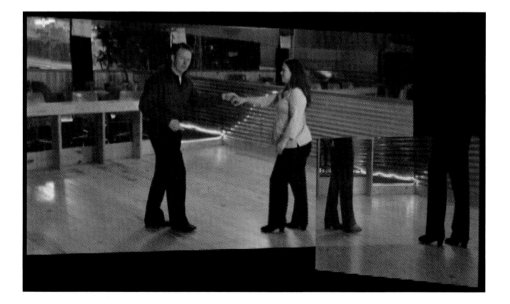

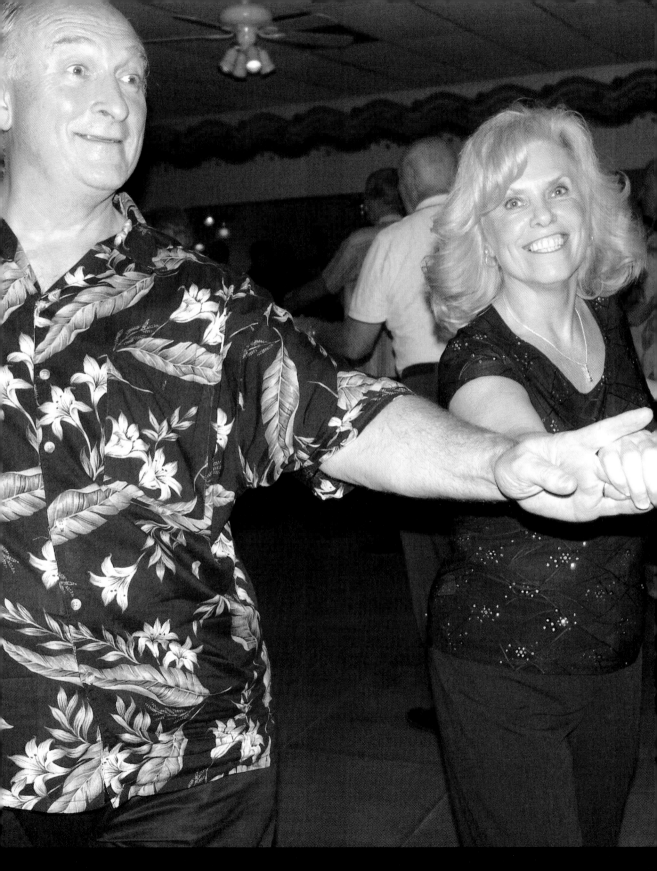

7

Picture Yourself
Dancing
Cha-Cha

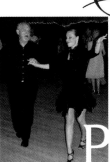

PICTURE YOURSELF moving confidently about the dance floor within the disciplined structure provided by the Latin dance that has a firm foothold in almost every genre of dance music, from Latin, to ballroom, to country, to today's Top 40 hits. In this chapter you will learn the basics and signature moves of a dance named for its signature step—the cha-cha-cha. Though the cha-cha is not a progressive dance, it is a dance of movement, with strong lateral motion coupled with forward and backward motion that can command a dance floor. The sensuous Latin motion, signature to all of the Latin dances, heats up the cha-cha from a strict-tempoed spot dance to a smoldering exhibition of rhythm and movement. Leaders, you'll assume the strong role appropriate to guide your partner to and fro across the dance floor, mastering the delicacy of the cha-cha while demonstrating the lead and follow skills integral to all couples dances. In the cha-cha, you will begin to experience independence from the closed dance frame and a follower with moves like chase turns and open breaks. You will be dancing one of the most popular Latin dances, one that has made a home in country-western nightclubs, ballroom studios, and of course the finest Latin clubs in the country.

The Six Ws of Cha-Cha

THE CHA-CHA, one of the youngest Latin dances to be introduced to the world of social dancing, has had a steady and growing following in Latin, country, and ballroom subcultures.

Who Created the Cha-Cha and Who Popularized It?

The cha-cha was created by dancers in Cuba. The dancers took aspects of the rumba and the mambo and danced the combination to slow mambo music.

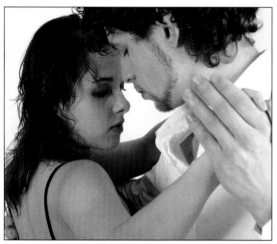

© istockphoto.com/Paul Piebinga

The cha-cha came to the United States via the ballroom community. While swing was sweeping the nation's popular culture, the ballrooms were looking to the South for inspiration. The ballroom instructors took and studied the cha-cha along with the other Latin dances and popularized them around the country and in Europe.

What Is the Cha-Cha?

The cha-cha is a dance born from the mambo. It was originally called the *triple mambo*, which then became the cha-cha-cha for the signature step. Eventually the name shortened to the cha-cha as we know it today. It is a spot dance to music of roughly 120 beats per minute.

> A *spot dance* describes any dance in which the partners dance for the most part in one "spot" on the floor. The dance basically centers on a central point, with the partners turning, changing directions, and rotating around that point.

It is an extremely smooth dance with a flirtatious and teasing tone with a very Latin sexy playfulness. Musically and rhythmically, the accent is on the second beat of every measure. The cha-cha is also marked by the traditional Latin motion and small, controlled steps taken on the ball of the foot. This disciplined technique creates a great deal of motion from the waist down, with a look as smooth as butter in the torso and above.

Where Did the Cha-Cha Originate and Where Is It Typically Done?

The cha-cha was born on the streets of Cuba to the rhythms of slow Caribbean mambo music. Because it is one of the most popular Latin dances, you can see and practice cha-cha at a wide variety of venues. Just as swing has made a home at almost every social event that involves dancing, cha-cha has found a beat in almost every genre of music from the '50s to today. Besides the traditional Caribbean music, many pop songs from yesterday and today also have the correct tempo and rhythmic structure for cha-cha. You will see cha-cha in ballrooms, in Latin nightclubs and country-western nightclubs, at social events such as weddings, reunions, and anniversaries, and on cruises as well as at resorts.

When Did the Cha-Cha Become Popular and When Is the Right Time to Cha-Cha?

The cha-cha has been described as the youngest of the Caribbean Latin dances, coming to light in the mid-1950s. Though cha-cha has never been a dance craze like its cousin, salsa, cha-cha has had a steady following in the ballroom world both nationally and internationally since its export from Cuba in the mid-twentieth century.

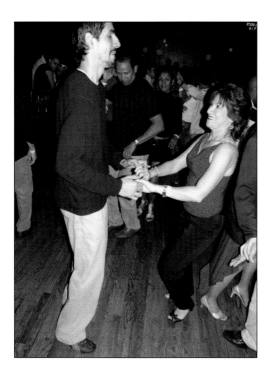

The right time to cha-cha can be described as any time you hear an appropriate song. If the song sounds like a cha-cha to you, get out on the dance floor and shake a leg. Other dancers might be doing West coast swing or a slow mambo, but don't let that inhibit you. Many times there are multiple dances that can accompany one song—a lot is determined by the tempo of the song. Just let your ears and your feet be your guide.

Why Is the Cha-Cha Danced?

As previously described, the cha-cha is a very flirtatious yet disciplined dance. It is a wonderful dance to showcase technique, form, and control. It is also a great dance for beginners to immerse themselves in because of the tight structure. Mistakes and problem areas are readily apparent and usually more fixable in the cha-cha than in dances that have a more casual and unstructured style. Also, because the cha-cha complements such a broad spectrum of musical selections and styles, it is a useful dance simply due to its versatility.

What Kind of Attire Should Be Worn?

There is no dress code or standard apparel for the cha-cha, and because you will see and dance the cha-cha in a wide variety of settings, it is most appropriate to dress for the occasion or venue. If you are going to a Latin club, the dress code is usually snappy and sassy nightclub attire, whereas if you are at a ballroom or other slightly more formal social event you might find yourself underdressed for the occasion.

Visualize the Cha-Cha

BEFORE STARTING the lesson plan for each dance, it's recommended that you take a few minutes or so to watch the DVD that accompanies this book and view the current section. In this case, you'll be watching the cha-cha segment to allow your mind's eye to start processing ideas on how to get your body to do what you're watching. Visualizing the cha-cha will give you a good feel for what you're about to learn and will make the transition into reality that much easier.

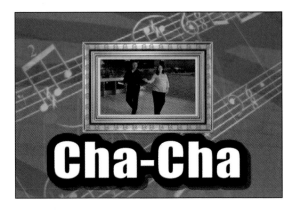

It's best if you watch the cha-cha section one time through without trying to do any of it. Just give your mind a chance to absorb the material so it's somewhat familiar to you when you hit replay to start the section over again. Watch how the dancers move, think about the words that are used, and picture yourself dancing the cha-cha.

The second time you watch the DVD, it's recommended that you take notes. Jot down the important parts of the cha-cha so you can engage other parts of the kinesthetic learning prior to getting up and dancing along. Write down what the connec-

tion points are, what the basic steps are called, how many counts are in a basic, how to align with your partner, and so on. Also, write down any questions that you might have about the cha-cha. There's a good chance you will find the answer later in this chapter, and if it's something you're already pondering, you'll be sure to remember the answer.

You'll find that by time you get ready to stand up and try the cha-cha with the DVD, the dancing won't be nearly as overwhelming. Writing down the key concepts will allow you to get a jumpstart on the rest of this chapter. You'll find that after you get up and try it, you'll probably have more questions. As this chapter goes on, the steps will be broken out with screenshots from the DVD, pointers will be given on where you should be during different parts of the dance, and frequently asked questions will be addressed that should satisfy most, if not all, of your questions and then some.

The third time you view the DVD, go ahead and dance along with it. See how far you can make it just by watching and trying. You'll probably find that one of the two of you is able to pick up and understand the material more quickly than the other.

> **Just remember, everyone learns at different paces. Be cognizant of this as you're learning with your partner. One of you might pick up certain aspects of the dance more quickly than the other, and that's okay. Try to be patient and wait for the other person to grasp the material, and then move on.**

Now, take a look at the rest of these pictures. All of them are taken of couples dancing the cha-cha. Some are formal, some are very informal, but they're all doing the same steps. See whether you can visualize yourself dancing the cha-cha (the dance you just watched over and over) in all these different settings. Then, picture yourself dancing the cha-cha at upcoming events or at local venues where you and your partner can go. Where will you go out dancing after you learn the cha-cha? Start thinking of the possibilities.

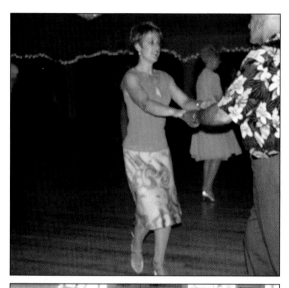

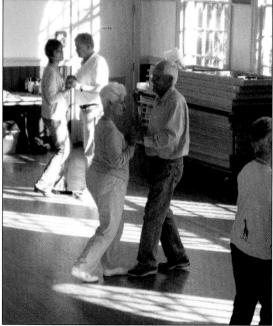

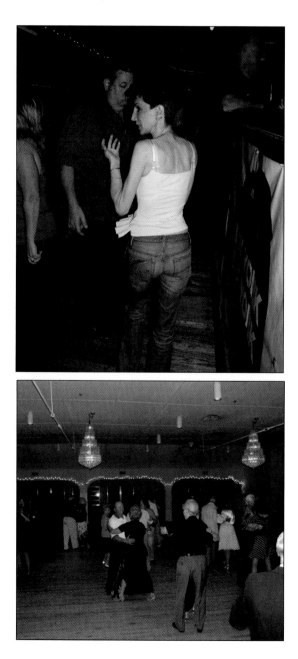

Cha-Cha Basics

C HA-CHA is best known for its strong lateral movements, and, of course, its trademark step, the cha-cha-cha! There are two main types of cha-cha, the American style and the international style. In a nutshell, it's most important to note that the difference lies mostly in the way the two are counted. Before we get into the basics, we'll talk about the two styles.

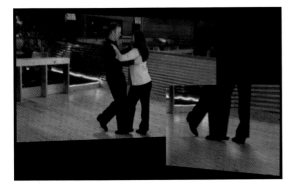

American style is counted using the phrase "cha-cha-cha," with which you might already be familiar. (Remember it used in the movie *Dirty Dancing*?) It sounds like this: one, two, cha-cha-cha, five, six, cha-cha-cha.

International style (which is also common in the United States) does not use the "cha-cha-cha" out loud in its basic count. Although the same steps are danced, they're danced to a different time in the music. The triple-step, or cha-cha-cha part of American style, is on counts three and four of the music, whereas the triple-step in international style is on the four and one or four and five of the music. It sounds like this: one, two, three, four-and-five, six, seven, eight-and-one.

> **Everything you learn in this chapter can easily be adapted to international style. The lead-and-follow portion will be identical, but the timing in the dance will change as mentioned previously. Leaders, we'll talk more about how to start the two different styles as we get further into the basics.**

As previously mentioned, the cha-cha is danced to 4/4 timing, which means the number of songs to practice with is quite extensive if you're just turning on your radio or pulling out your CD or MP3 collection. For specific songs or up-to-date playlists, it might be best to do a search online for "cha-cha music" and find a few songs from whatever genre of music is your favorite, and then practice along. You should familiarize yourself with the cool cha-cha beat and with the timing in order to recognize the dance when the opportunity arises. Before we begin the cha-cha, let's touch on our two most important rules:

1. Ladies are always right! Ladies, put your weight on your left foot so you can be ready to start with your right. (This is what's called your *ready position*.)

2. Guys always get what's left. Guys, put your weight on your right foot so you can be ready to start with your left. (This is what's called your *ready position*.)

The Eight-Count Basic

Cha-cha uses a slow, slow, quick-quick-slow rhythm where the slows are considered *break-steps* because the partners "break away" from each other. The break-steps are also commonly called *rock-steps*, which is how we will refer to them for our purposes in this text. The quick-quick-slow is a *triple-step*, which is the signature "cha-cha-cha" step of the dance. The eight-count basic of cha-cha is made up of two sets of rock-steps and triple-steps. Essentially, it's called out: one, two, cha-cha-cha, five, six, cha-cha-cha. The rock-steps are on the counts one, two, and again on five, six. Triple-steps are what make up the cha-cha-cha and are found on the counts three-and-four and again on seven-and-eight.

The dance starts with the leaders rocking forward and followers rocking back on count one. Count two lets both partners finish the rock-step portion and put their weight onto the original foot. For the counts three-and-four, you'll do a triple-step in place and call it cha-cha-cha. (You could also say this as quick-quick-slow.) You're now through with half of the basic. The other half is the exact opposite.

On count five, leaders will now rock back while the followers are rocking forward, and on six, both partners will replace their weight and finish the rock-step. Counts seven-and-eight are the same as three-and-four, just with the opposite foot, because they are the cha-cha-cha portion to end the basic.

> **Cha-cha-cha is the equivalent of a triple-step, or quick-quick-slow, where the quicks are half a beat and the slows are a whole beat.**

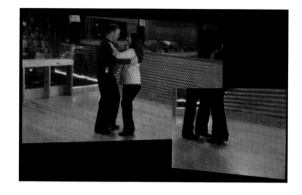

Cha-cha, in layman's terms, is said out loud like this:

Rock-step, cha-cha-cha, rock-step, cha-cha-cha,

Rock-step, cha-cha-cha, rock-step, cha-cha-cha

If you're more mathematically inclined and like to use numbers for your steps, it's counted like this:

One, two, three-and-four, five, six, seven-and-eight,

One, two, three-and-four, five, six, seven-and-eight

Cha-cha also incorporates what's called *Latin motion*, or *Cuban motion*. Because the styling for the cha-cha is flirtatious in nature, it's easy to picture what this motion should look like. For the right look and feel of Latin motion, you must use your knees rather than your hips, but it's not easy. Latin motion is a direct result of bending one knee slightly while the other straightens, and then vice versa. This means that when you step, you'll use the ball of your foot first, then your heel, almost as if you're digging into the ground.

Turn your toes in slightly to keep your knees from separating too much and to give the impression that your knees are working together rather than just opening up. This is something to practice to achieve the right look as you continue to practice your basics and add new moves to your cha-cha repertoire.

Basics in Place

To try the cha-cha basics in place (you can stand next to one another for this one), assume foot position 1 and be in your respective ready positions. Next, you'll want to simply rock on count one (changing weight), then step down on count two (again changing weight). Guys, you'll be rocking forward, and ladies will be rocking backward. (Remember, your steps are opposite.) Then, you'll both do the triple-step in place (cha-cha-cha), then you'll rock the other direction. (If you rocked forward first, now you'll rock back, and vice versa.) This same pattern will now take you through the eight-count basic, so after you've done it once, go ahead and repeat it over and over just for fun. Doing this a few times should get you familiar with the timing and the changing of weight. At the end of every eight counts, you should be ready to start back over on count one with your first rock-step. And yes, at the end of each basic (when you're doing them in place), you'll be in your ready position, so just keep that in mind as you go through each one.

Mirroring: Left and Right Basics

When you're comfortable with the basics, go ahead and move into the next section, which allows you to do the full basics of the cha-cha without having

to worry about anything but the footwork. For learning your individual steps the first time, stand directly in front of each other (slightly offset). Rather than just doing the basics in place, this time we're going to move with them. Try facing each other as shown in the figure below, but be about two to five feet away from your partner in a mirrored position. It often helps if you're able to see the opposite steps, if for no other reason than to validate your own.

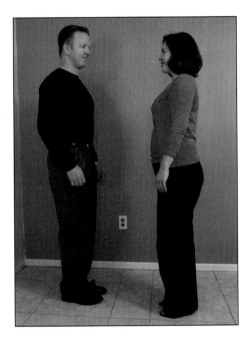

1. (Step 1 - Count 1) From a ready position, leaders will rock forward with their left foot (fourth foot position), and followers will rock back with their right foot (also in fourth foot position), with each partner changing weight to the foot that was moving by the end of step or count 1.

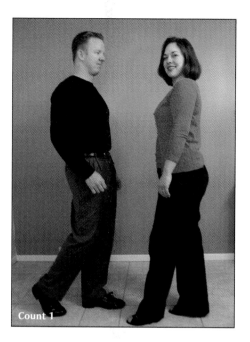

Count 1

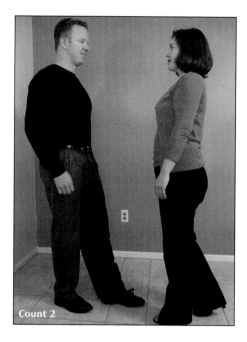

Count 2

2. (Step 2 - Count 2) Leaders, shift your weight back onto your right foot as you complete the "step" portion of the rock-step (fourth foot position). Followers, shift your weight forward onto your left foot as you complete the "step" portion of the rock-step (fourth foot position).

3. (Steps 3, 4, 5 - Counts 3 and 4) Leaders, step with your left foot to the left into a second foot position on count 3, bring your right foot together on the count "and" (first foot position), then step left again into a second foot position to your left on count 4. This cha-cha-cha portion will now have you traveling to your left as you face your partner. Followers, step with your right foot to the right into a second foot position on count 3, bring your left foot together on the count "and" (first foot position), then step right again into a second foot position to your right on count 4. The exact opposite of the

guys, this cha-cha-cha portion will now have you traveling to your right as you face your partner.

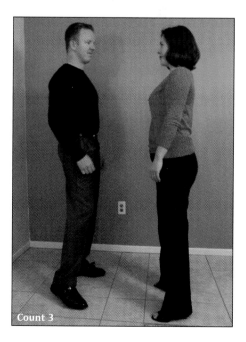

Count 3

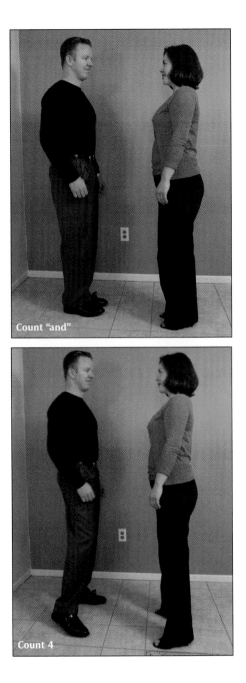

Count "and"

Count 4

slow down a little. With your right foot, you'll now start your rock-step back with the "rock" portion. Your weight will now be directly over your right foot in a rocking manner, and your left foot will remain in front (suspended in air) in fourth foot position. Followers, you're now on your right foot and your momentum has also kicked in, so you, too, must slow down a little and gain control. With your left foot, you'll now start your rock-step as you step forward for the "rock." Your weight is directly over your left foot, and your right foot is slightly elevated, yet it's still in fourth foot position.

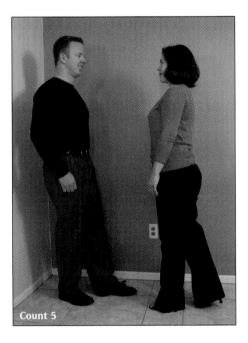

Count 5

4. (Step 6 - Count 5) Leaders, you're now on your left foot and you've got to stop your momentum in order to take the next step, so

5. (Step 7 - Count 6) Leaders, you're now rocking backward on your right foot and you've got to shift your weight forward to your left. Completing the rock-step, you'll step onto your left foot (still in fourth foot position) and place your weight firmly on top of it. Followers, you're on your left foot and you'll

be finishing the rock-step by stepping back onto your right foot. Upon completion, you'll be standing directly on top of your right foot (and in fourth foot position).

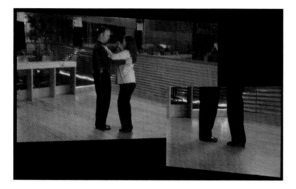

6. (Steps 8, 9, 10 - Counts 7 and 8) Leaders, step with your right foot to the right into a second foot position on count 7, bring your left foot together on the count "and" (first foot position), then step right again into a second foot position to your right on count 8. This cha-cha-cha portion will now have you traveling to your right as you face your partner and complete your basic. Followers, step with your left foot to the left into a second foot position on count 7, bring your right foot together on the count "and" (first foot position), then step left again into a second foot position to your left on count 8. The exact opposite of the guy's footwork, this

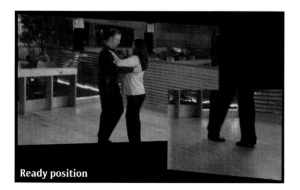

Ready position

cha-cha-cha portion will now have you traveling to your left as you face your partner and complete your basic.

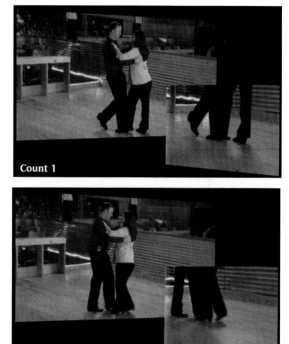

Count 1

Count 2

As soon as you're both able to do the basics from side to side over and over and over again (correctly), go ahead and practice with music.

> **As you do the basic footwork, be sure to keep your rock-steps under control. If either partner takes too large of a step back or forward in the rock-step, it will throw you off beat and you might end up stepping on your partner.**

Leaders, count out loud to give the follower a chance to match you step for step when you start. The leader should say "Ready, go" or "Ready, and" on counts 5 and 7 (the equivalent of slow, slow) just prior to starting. The 5 and 7 here refer to the music that you're listening to as you prepare to take your first step. Think of the old dance movies in which they give a countdown of "5-6-7-8" before starting. This is the same thing, but because you'll be starting with slows, it's best to start in on that timing, just like you would in swing. To start, it'd be like this: "Ready, and" slow, slow or one, two. This should make it easier for both partners.

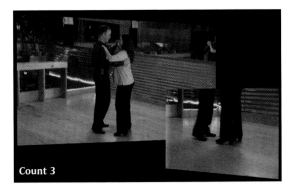

Count 3

As always, if either partner gets on the "wrong foot" during the exercise, just stop, laugh, and start up again after the leader counts it off. . . "Ready, and," and you're back dancing again.

Practice until you're both comfortable with the steps and the answers to each of the following questions:

▶ **At the end of each basic, should you be in your ready position or in second foot position?**

▶ **Are there any steps that you'll take in an eight-count basic that do not include a change of weight?**

▶ **How many steps are taken in the eight-count basic?**

▶ **What are the foot positions typically used for the rock-steps in cha-cha?**

▶ **How many triple-steps are taken in the eight-count basic by each partner?**

The Eight-Count Basic as a Couple

Are you an expert on the basics? Are you ready to dance with someone other than your shadow? Okay then, it's time to put your body into the game and not just let your feet have all the fun. If you've practiced the basics enough on your own, you'll be able to focus on just the new material that's about to be introduced. Leaders, this is especially important for you because you don't want to be learning to lead at the same time as you're learning your steps. If you skipped right to this section and didn't practice it on your own, you might have a tough time figuring out where any problems are if they arise. Practicing before coming together is a critical building block; the confidence each partner brings makes it much easier because you'll both have high expectations. As repeated throughout this book, social dancing is close to 25-percent skill and 75-percent attitude, so keep up the great work you've been doing and the positive comments toward your partner.

Your toolkit for the cha-cha basics includes:

▶ **Foot position 1 (ready position, and on the two "and" steps; in other words, 3 and 4 as well as 7 and 8)**

▶ **Foot position 2 (counts 3, 4, 7, 8 of the basic)**

▶ **Foot position 4 (counts 1, 2, 5, 6 of the basic)**

▶ **Connection points 1–4 (all will be used here in the basic)**

▶ **Eight-count basic (essential for the cha-cha to work)**

Go ahead and get into your dance position (all four connection points), and let's start the cha-cha. Now that your frame is set up, your feet are offset, and you're in your ready position, let's give it a shot. Ready? Leaders, go ahead and give your starting count of "Ready, and," then rock forward and back, then do your triple-step to the side with your left, and then rock back and forward and finish with your triple to the right. Now that you got through one basic, just repeat it over and over. How 'bout that? You're now doing the basics of cha-cha. . .rock-step, cha-cha-cha, rock-step, cha-cha-cha, (and again!) rock-step, cha-cha-cha, rock-step, cha-cha-cha. . . . Hooray!

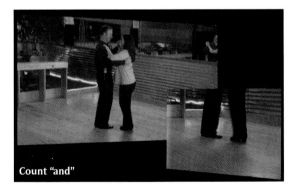

Count "and"

Are you comfortable with it? If so, and you're both feeling good about your progress, turn your attention to the lead-and-follow portion of the dance. This way, you'll ensure that both of you understand what all is happening and how it's all broken down. Just as you've had to in many other dances, you've got a lot to put together here to make it all

work. The cha-cha basic can be broken into four logical pieces, each consisting of its own unique lead-and-follow aspects. Next, we'll look at each of these pieces in depth in the hopes of conveying a complete and thorough understanding to you. Once you understand these pieces from the "basic" perspective, you'll be able to apply them to every move you do, so make sure you spend the time going through each one.

Part 1

Leaders, to leave your partner with no doubts as you start your dance, you'll first want to lean toward her from a closed dance position, almost as if you're tipping forward. You'll do this lean somewhere around counts 7 or 8 of the "5-6-7-8" countdown prior to starting the dance. Because you're both in your ready positions, this lean will now put your bodies in motion in order to start the rock-step on counts 1-2.

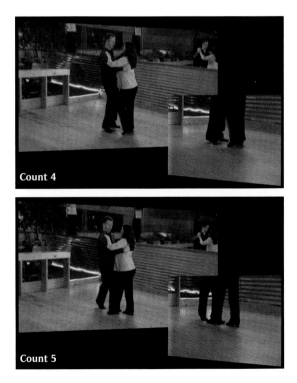

Count 4

Count 5

Followers, it's essential to have your connection point 4 in place in order to feel the leader's body heading your direction. Even more so, you should feel a combination of connection points 4 and 1 coming toward you, which is your first clue to get out of the way by leaning back. At the same time, connection point 2 will be shifting slightly backward to let you move back and away from your partner as you maintain your frame.

> If the followers don't move out of the way or lean back when the leaders are coming toward them, it's quite possible that the leader will smash into the follower in an unpleasant manner. Unless this is the follower's objective, it's best to use the clues that are provided.

Next, on the rock-step, the leaders must also take control and ensure that the follower's weight doesn't continue going backward. (Remember, that's where the momentum is headed.) Connection point 2 will now be used by the leaders because their right hand must now gradually slow the momentum down on the "rock" (almost as if to catch the follower in their right hand). After slowing the momentum (almost to a complete stop after the follower is firmly on her right foot), connection point 2 will be used to change the direction of the follower's body.

Going into the "step" portion of the rock-step, the leader will now use his right hand to control the follower by gently shifting her weight forward onto her left foot. Although the right hand (connection point 2) is the primary lead, it doesn't work by itself. The shifting of weight here is a fallout of the leader's weight shifting back onto his right foot and his frame coming with him. Everything works together, but connection point 2 is the one that makes or breaks this portion because it has the lead role in bringing the follower along.

Followers, you should feel as though your body is being slowed down and then redirected without giving you whiplash. If it feels rough at all, have the leader continue working on it until it's smooth. It should almost be so smooth that you don't even realize that your body momentum has changed. (This means it has to be gradual, guys!) As soon as the transition has taken place, you should be evenly weighted over your left foot and ready to step with your right foot.

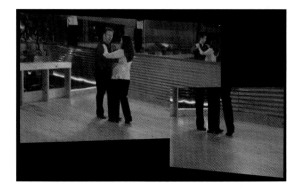

Part 2

Leaders, this is where you take this dance from one direction to the next. You're now going to take your partner to your left with a clear, deliberate motion that gives her no choice. After you've finished the rock-step and you're firmly on your right foot and she's up and on her left, you'll start your movement to the side. In doing so, connection points 1 and 2 are going to share in the "lead role," while connection points 3 and 4 will be cast as supporting roles only. Although it shares in the lead role on this step, connection point 1 is pretty much in charge of keeping the follower's body aligned with yours as you move it out to your left.

Connection point 2 will make or break the side-steps. Leaders, the palm of your right hand (you could also use the wrist area of your right arm as a guide) is in charge of redirecting the follower's weight and sending it to the side. The connection must be solid, and the follower must feel as though you're in complete control of her body.

> **Leaders, go ahead and try this one out for a moment. Have the follower stand on her left foot while you're in closed dance position, and see what it takes to get her to move to her right (your left). All you have to do here is move directly to the side and get her to step with her right foot while still facing you. (Remember, connection point 1 helps with the alignment.)**

Followers, you should feel unable to step anywhere but to your right side, and your frame should keep you directly in line with the leader. The pressure that you feel on your left shoulder blade should be constant, rather than a digging, poking, or even a sharp nudge. Everything should be smooth here as your body transitions from one direction to the next. Indicators of something going wrong would include you not being aligned with your partner (basically squared up, although offset), your head being thrown to one side or the other, or you feeling uncomfortable with the lead from connection point 2. If it's right, you should barely feel a thing, yet you'll be in the correct position at the end of it.

Back to the leaders here for a moment. Leaders, now that you've successfully redirected your partner, you need to keep the momentum up and do the triple-step here in the middle, or the cha-cha-cha. It's essential that you keep your body aligned

with your partner while you're moving her to the side. Don't falter on the direction; it really needs to be the same throughout counts 3 and 4. The side cha-cha-cha portion will put both yours and your partner's feet into the second foot position on the first cha, then the first foot position on the second cha (the "and" step), and finally, back to the second foot position for the final cha.

> **An easy way to remember and practice the side-steps is to say "side-together-side" in place of "cha-cha-cha."**

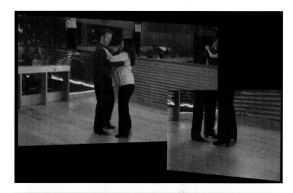

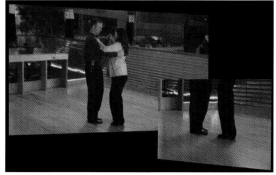

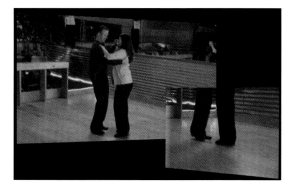

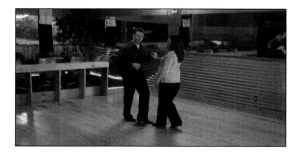

Part 3

Part 3 of the basic is very similar to Part 1, except it reverses what was done. For the leaders, instead of rocking forward and then back, you'll now be rocking back and then forward (and it'll be with a different foot). By the time you finish the first cha-cha-cha, leaders, you'll be on your left foot and ready to step with your right. As such, you're now going to do the "rock" portion of the rock-step, starting back with your right foot. Followers, as you can imagine, as the leader rocks back with his right foot, you'll be rocking forward with your left.

Leaders, to get the follower to rock forward with her left foot, you have to change her direction again. No longer will you be going to the side because you'll now have to get her to rock toward you. First things first: In order to stop the momentum, connection point 1 basically puts up a roadblock at the end of the cha-cha-cha, and connection point 2 stops "pushing to the side."

Now, leaders, your connection point 2 has to bring the follower's left shoulder blade toward you as you shift the right side of your body back while en route to do your rock-step. By shifting the follower's shoulder blade toward you, you'll cause her weight to shift and the need for her to step forward.

Followers, you should feel just enough of a pull here on your left shoulder blade (connection point 2), that you have no choice but to step forward. It shouldn't be so strong that it feels like you're being yanked forward, but it does have to be enough to get you to step.

Now, once you've both taken the rock, connection point 4 comes into play (along with connection point 1). Leaders, you now have to head back toward your partner with a nice, easy shifting of your weight forward in the attempt to get back onto your left foot to do the "step" portion of the rock-step. Although it happens quickly, everything still has to take place to pull it off without a hitch. Followers, you should feel your partner now coming toward you, and you should feel connection points 1 and 4 giving you clues to shift your weight backward (or else!). By the end of this rock-step, leaders should be firmly on their left foot, ready to step with their right, and followers should be on their right foot, ready to step with their left.

Part 4

Part 4 of the basic is the exact opposite of Part 2. Leaders, you'll be moving your partners to your right instead of your left. The cha-cha-cha portion (or side-together-side) is the exact opposite; both partners will step into the second foot position, then into first, then back into second (leaders step to their right and followers step to their left).

Leaders, you'll find that the easiest and most effi-cient way to move your partner to the left will be with a combination of connection point 1 and the finger portion of connection point 2 (as if to "pull" off to the right). Connection point 1 will provide the pressure (almost a slight push) to the leader's right to get the follower to step off to her left. At the same time that there's pushing with one side of the body, there's pulling with the other (connec-tion point 2) because they both have to work together.

Followers, the lead here should be transparent to you—you should just feel your body moving to the left. You shouldn't feel pushed on one side or pulled on the other. Tell the leader when it feels right and also whether something needs to change, because he might not be aware of how hard or how light he's being with you. At the end of the cha-cha-cha portion (the last cha), though, you should feel your momentum slowing down almost to a stop again, because connection point 2 should keep you from moving any farther.

It's now time to put the entire basic together with each of the four parts. Remember, once you under-stand the dynamics of each of these leads, you'll be able to use them in additional moves. They won't be just for the basics. Your goal for now is to get through the basics and make them look and feel natural. Guys, the more you understand how to manipulate the woman's momentum and motion through nonverbal leads, the better off you'll be. Ladies, the more you know about what feels right and why, the better you'll be in following because you'll know how to compensate when needed and you'll know when to just sit back and enjoy the dance.

Go ahead and dance through the cha-cha basics a few times. Is it working? Go through this next list and talk about what happened to you (good or bad) as you attempted the cha-cha.

▶ **You successfully completed all eight counts (each time).**

▶ **You felt completely overwhelmed with all the details of the basic.**

▶ **You managed to stay directly in front of your partner (slightly offset).**

▶ **You felt a bit uncoordinated, yet more enlightened for going through it.**

▶ **You were smiling or caused your partner to smile with your perplexed look.**

▶ **You're optimistic because you feel as though you're getting better with each try.**

To recap this one, there are several different leads going on during the cha-cha basic. As usual, the follower should feel as though her body is com-pletely controlled by the leader. There should be enough of a lead that the follower could literally do the steps blindfolded.

Practicing with the follower blindfolded (or at least closing her eyes) is a great way to practice and to test the leader's command of the dance as well as the follower's reception. The fact that the follower is blindfolded should have no impact on the couple's success on the dance floor. She should be able to do every step without using her eyes. This practicing tool works for any of the couples dances.

Obviously, the more time you spend on the basics, the better off you'll be. If there's a part you don't understand or one that just simply isn't working, you might want to contact a local professional to get it worked out. Success is marked when everything is working together and both partners are moving effortlessly with one another.

When you're able to do the basics over and over without problems, you'll be ready to put it all together with the next page full of fun drills. We're going to add in a number of variations in the drills for you to work further with the rock-step, cha-cha-cha rhythm. See whether you can follow along as we go, because this is where your thinking skills will come into play. Have fun!

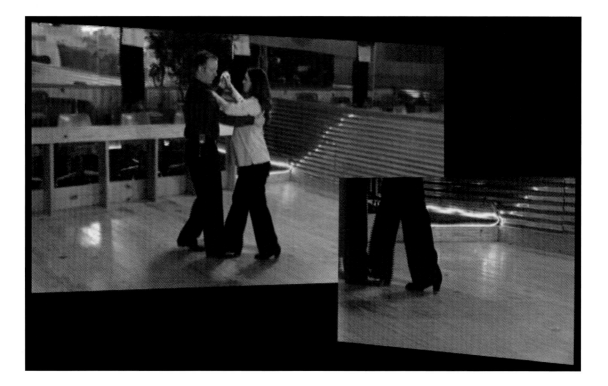

Fun Drills to Put It All Together

JUST LIKE AT THE END of every dance, we've put together several fun drills and exercises for you to go through to work on your cha-cha. Instead of just picturing yourself doing the cha-cha, it's time to put it all together and add on. Go through each drill as they focus on different moves, leads, and thinking patterns. Soon, you'll feel confident enough to dance the cha-cha in front of almost anyone.

Drill 1: Shadow Dancing

Set up in your ready position in your dance frame, but do the basics on your own. Have your partner do theirs as well, just not with you because they'll be a couple of feet away. Turn some music on and dance through each of the four parts repetitively. See who can last the longest without messing up, stopping, or getting off beat.

Drill 2: The Tortoise and the Hare

Set up in your ready position, but this time with your partner, and test several different speeds of the cha-cha. No music is necessary, but it helps if you have it because you'll have fun practicing slow speed, normal speed (you'll decide what normal is), and then as fast as you can handle.

Drill 3: Progressive Basics

Rather than doing the basics with a rock-step and then to the side before repeating, you're now going to try the basics straight forward and back.

Leaders, as soon as you're finished with the rock-step on counts 1, 2, you're going to travel straight backward while doing the cha-cha-cha. To make it work, leaders, you *cannot* deviate or even hint at the fact that you're going to go sideways—just take your partner straight back with you as you pass your feet while doing your cha-cha-cha. Just after the first cha-cha-cha, leaders, you'll do your rock-step straight back with your right foot. (Followers, you'll be rocking forward with your left.) Then, leaders, do your cha-cha-cha steps directly toward your partner as you have her moving backward. The timing on this drill is the exact same, and you can go back into your regular basics at any point. Doing progressive basics just gives you more of a variety as you work on the essential pieces of the cha-cha.

Drill 4: Two, One, Zero

As an add-on to Drill 3 (while doing the progressive basics), leaders can drop from the closed dance position into a two-hand hold (with their hands underneath and in control—just their thumbs would be on top). After a couple of times, try going from a two-hand hold into a one-hand hold (it can be either hand as long as there's still a lead). You can also do the progressive basics with no hands at all because the lead is strictly visual, yet the steps are the same. This is the start of what's called a *chase-turn*, which is done from an open progressive. Try all three of these together and see how you like them. You can then try them all with your regular basic, and it'll add quite a variety.

Hot Tips for the Cha-Cha

S A COOL AND CLASSY dance, the cha-cha has some definite styling differences that need to be pointed out. Following are a number of tips, pointers, and reminders for dancing the cha-cha now that you're feeling good about the basics and ready to move forward. Keep each one in mind as you practice your dance out there on the floor.

▶ **Small, controlled steps are best as you learn and get familiar with the basics.**

▶ **Soft knees are important for an overall relaxed look and to develop the starting point for your Latin or Cuban motion.**

▶ **Change weight! In cha-cha, your steps should be clearly defined and should not consist of a shuffle or a bounce. Most importantly, each step must contain a transfer of weight.**

▶ **Having fun on the dance floor is more important than being technically correct on everything but not enjoying it.**

▶ **Avoid shaking or twisting your hips in the attempt to have Latin or Cuban motion. The correct Latin motion is a direct result of the feet, knees, and legs; however, if you don't have the steps or the leading/following aspects down, Latin motion isn't going to do anything for your dance.**

▶ **Don't bounce! Cha-cha is a very rhythmic dance, but it doesn't have a vertical (up and down) look to it. The dance should be very smooth and controlled.**

▶ **It takes eight beats to dance one full cha-cha basic. The basic can be danced either front and back or side to side. Either one works and has its own particular lead-and-follow elements to it.**

▶ **The cha-cha basics are the most important. Do them well, and you'll be able to do almost anything out on the social dance floor. Practice them until they become second nature.**

▶ **Keep your head up, your partner slightly offset, and your frame intact. Shoot for the look of confidence and relaxation, regardless of what all is going on inside your head.**

▶ **The difference between American- and international-style cha-cha is how the dance starts and what count the rock-steps (a.k.a. break-steps) occur. To dance international style, leaders first take a side-step to their left on count 1, then do the rock-step on 2, 3, the side cha-cha-cha steps on 4 and 5, the rock-steps again on 6, 7, then the cha-cha-cha portion again on 8 and 1 (the 1 starts the next basic).**

▶ **Cha-cha should be fun and sexy, so dance it that way.**

Review and Next Steps for Your Cha-Cha

ALL RIGHT, ANOTHER chapter down and "in the books!" Let's do a final recap here and make sure you're comfortable with the major concepts and points of the cha-cha. Go through each one and come back to this list as necessary for a quick review.

Review

1. Ladies are always right! Ladies, put your weight on your left foot so you can be ready to start with your right. (In other words, get in your ready position.)

2. Guys always get what's left. Guys, put your weight on your right foot so you can be ready to start with your left. (In other words, get in your ready position.)

3. All four connection points are used in the basics of the cha-cha (whether to the side or progressive). If you're doing progressive basics, remember that you can also do them with just connection point 1 (single-hand hold or two-hand hold), or without any connection points in a mirrored fashion.

4. The cha-cha basic consists of eight counts (rock-step, cha-cha-cha, rock-step, cha-cha-cha) and is more important than any other step because it's the one you'll be repeating over and over and over.

5. American style and international style differ mainly in the placement of the rock-step within an eight-count measure of music. In American style, you rock (or break) on the 1, 2, then also on the 5, 6; whereas in international style you rock on the 2, 3 and also on the 6, 7. Be flexible and versatile by knowing both styles.

6. Rock-steps are primarily done in fourth foot position when starting out with the basics. Gradually, as your Latin motion improves, you might find yourself somewhere between the fourth and fifth foot positions when you rock.

7. The basics consist of four separate parts, and each one is led and followed a bit differently. The first part is the initial rock-step, then the second is the first cha-cha-cha, then the rock-step the other direction, and finally the second cha-cha-cha that takes you back to your beginning.

Next Steps

Upon mastering the mystery of the cha-cha, including all its stylings, you might find that you're ready for more. Whether it's more about leading, following, additional moves and patterns, Latin motion, or just the basics, there are plenty of places to learn. Local ballroom dance studios are the best places to look for competent instruction as a starting point, but you can always do a quick online search to find community dance classes that might provide you with what you need. Cha-cha is a great dance to have in your back pocket because you'll be ready to dance in almost every setting. Put on a nice pair of threads and go out there and show the world that you've got skills!

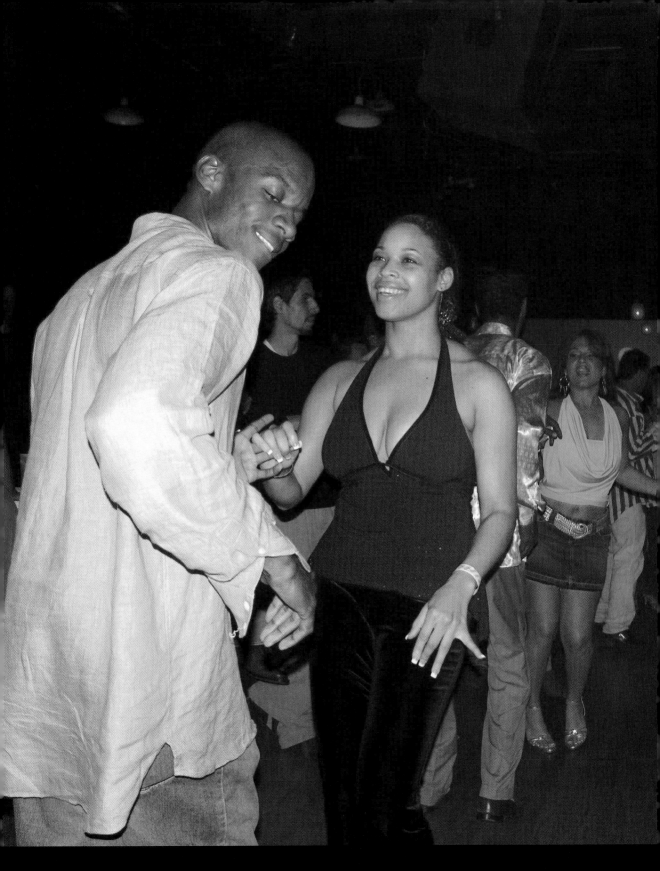

8

Picture Yourself

Dancing

Salsa

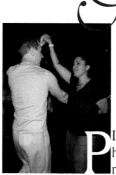

PICTURE YOURSELF on a sultry evening in the hottest Latin club on the strip. You and your partner, whether or not you are of Latin heritage, are burning up the floor to the hot salsa beat. As you master the basics of the salsa, you are attaining proficiency in a very fast dance that combines the trademark Latin motion with quick footwork, strong leads, and a combination of both open and closed dance positions. If you are the leader, you are holding the baseline of the salsa beat with your footwork while you guide your partner through a variety of moves, all led seamlessly and seemingly effortlessly. As the follower, you appear to be hovering above the floor; the rapid footwork and Latin motion create optical illusions because most of the rapid action is seen from the waist down. Your relaxed demeanor as your partner guides you through various moves disguises all of the activity necessary to execute this spicy dance. As one of the hottest dances to gain popularity in mainstream couples dancing since the swing, you will see and dance salsa at more and more locations and functions. Once only danced in Latin nightclubs, you will now see yourself dancing salsa at weddings, parties, and other social occasions, much the way you see swing dancing at these events.

The Six Ws of Salsa

SALSA IS AS EXCITING and spicy a dance as its name. Unlike some of the other dances, salsa has stayed remarkably close to its roots and has not been drastically adapted for the greater dancing public, unlike tango and swing.

Who Created the Salsa and Who Popularized It?

Though not named in Cuba, the dance and music were born there and grew into the salsa that we know today through the influences of Cuban, Puerto Rican, and Afro-Caribbean music.

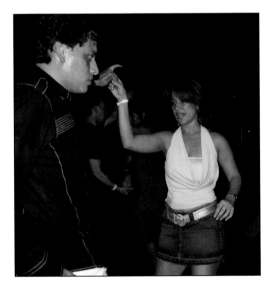

The Latin American community can be credited with the distinctive style, name, and ever-growing popularity of salsa. Over the last few years, salsa has become one of the most popular dances for beginner social dancers to learn, rivaling the swing in size of following.

What Is the Salsa?

The name "salsa" was given to the blended Puerto Rican and Cuban dance music that emerged when the immigrants began mixing the music and dance styles of their home islands. Salsa, meaning "sauce," describes the mixture of instrumentation, vocal arrangement, and percussion that are key ingredients for any salsa song. Such a variety of percussion instruments are used that it is sometimes difficult for beginners to identify the underlying beat of the song! Though the timing for salsa is the same as every other popular song today (4/4), with the exception of waltz, salsa music is obvious to even the untrained ear the minute it begins. Salsa is an eight-count spot dance that has its roots in the mambo. The basic beat distribution and foot movement patterns are the same, but the styling and overall look are quite different.

A *spot dance* describes any dance in which the partners dance for the most part in one "spot" on the floor. The dance basically centers on a central point, with the partners turning, changing directions, and rotating around that point.

Salsa is a smooth dance, meaning there is little, if any, up and down motion of the dance partners as they move. Almost all of the action is from the waist down, and from the waist down, the dancers are smokin'! Salsa music for the most part is very fast—the slower end of the spectrum of salsa music is more appropriately matched to cha-cha. Though good control of the dancer's body is necessary for a successful salsa, the key to greatness is found in getting into the hot and spicy feel of the dance and truly enjoying the music and movement.

Where Did Salsa Originate and Where Is It Typically Done?

Salsa as we know it today, a separate dance from the mambo, originated in New York City, in the neighborhoods largely populated by Latin Caribbean immigrants.

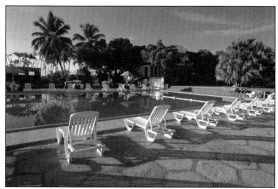
© istockphoto.com/Steven Miric

Because salsa is still growing in popularity, you will see it and dance it at a growing number of venues. You can learn and dance salsa at a ballroom, but this is a more structured and formal version of the dance, adapted to the regimented syllabi that allow ballrooms to standardize dances for competition and instruction purposes. Freestyle salsa is most commonly seen in salsa nightclubs, though you will see it at more and more social events, Latin and otherwise, as the dance continues to gain popularity.

When Did the Salsa Become Popular and When Is the Right Time to Salsa?

Salsa was born in the 1960s in New York as a distinct music and dance style from mambo and cha-cha. Salsa has attained renewed and greater popularity in recent years through publicity associated with several popular movies.

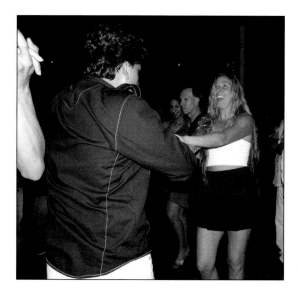

The right time to salsa is any time you hear the music. Because salsa is a spot dance, it doesn't require much space—the dance floor at most salsa nightclubs is so crowded you wonder how anyone has space to catch a breath! Because salsa music is so distinctive and specialized for dancing, the mere playing of salsa music is usually a call to dance. Just let your ears and your feet be your guides.

Why Is the Salsa Danced?

As previously described, salsa is a very spicy and sexy, yet disciplined, dance. It is a wonderful dance to "let loose" and celebrate the art and sensation of couples dancing as a whole. It is also a great dance for beginners to immerse themselves in due to the simple footwork and beat pattern. The repetitive nature of the foot pattern is like a security blanket as a dancer learns moves. Though salsa is spicy and sexy, it is also a dance that celebrates movement and music, and is a wonderful addition to any dancer's repertoire.

What Kind of Attire Should Be Worn?

There is no dress code or standard apparel for the salsa, and because you will see and dance salsa in a few different settings, it is most appropriate to dress for the occasion or venue. If you are going to a Latin club, the dress code is usually snappy and sassy nightclub attire, whereas if you are at a ballroom or other slightly more formal social event, you might find yourself underdressed in your club attire.

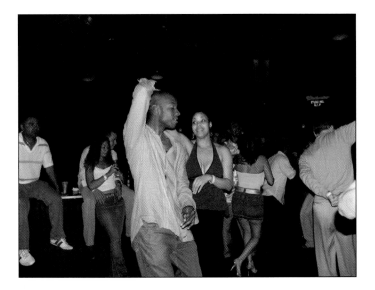

Visualize the Salsa

BEFORE STARTING the lesson plan for each dance, it's recommended you take a few minutes or so to watch the DVD that accompanies this book and view the current section. In this case, you'll be watching the salsa segment to allow your mind's eye to start processing ideas for how to get your body to do what you're watching. Visualizing the salsa will give you a good feel for what you're about to learn and will make the transition into reality that much easier.

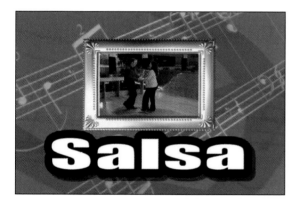

It's best if you watch the salsa section one time through without trying to do any of it. Just give your mind a chance to absorb the material so it's somewhat familiar to you when you hit replay to start the section over again. Watch how the dancers move, think about the words that are used, and picture yourself dancing the salsa.

The second time you watch the DVD, it's recommended that you take notes. Jot down the important parts of the salsa so you can engage other parts of the kinesthetic learning prior to getting up and dancing along. Write down what the connection points are, what the basic steps are called,

how many counts are in a basic, how to align with your partner, and so on. Also, write down any questions that you might have about the salsa. There's a good chance you will find the answer later in this chapter, and if it's something you're already pondering, you'll be sure to remember the answer.

You'll find that by the time you get ready to stand up and try the salsa with the DVD, the dancing won't be nearly as overwhelming. Writing down the key concepts will allow you to get a jumpstart on the rest of this chapter. You'll find that after you get up and try it, you'll probably have more questions. As this chapter goes on, the steps will be broken out with screenshots from the DVD, pointers will be given on where you should be during different parts of the dance, and frequently asked questions will be addressed that should satisfy most, if not all, of your questions and then some.

The third time you view the DVD, go ahead and dance along with it. See how far you can make it just by watching and trying. You'll probably find that one of the two of you is able to pick up and understand the material more quickly than the other.

> **Just remember, everyone learns at different paces. Be cognizant of this as you're learning with your partner. One of you might pick up certain aspects of the dance quicker than the other, and that's okay. Try to be patient and wait for the other person to grasp the material, and then move on.**

Now, take a look at the rest of these pictures. All of them are taken of couples dancing the salsa. Some are formal, some are very informal, but they're all doing the same steps. See whether you can visualize yourself dancing salsa (the dance you just watched over and over) in all these different settings. Then, picture yourself dancing salsa at upcoming events or at local venues where you and your partner can go. Where will you go out dancing after you learn the salsa? Start thinking of the possibilities and get ready for a good time!

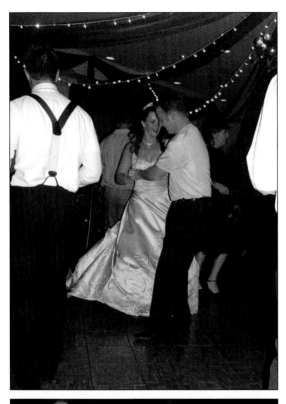

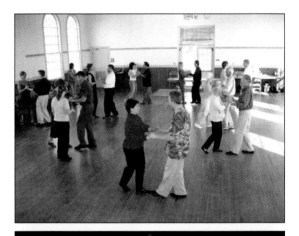

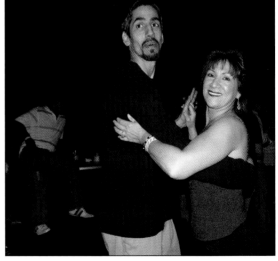

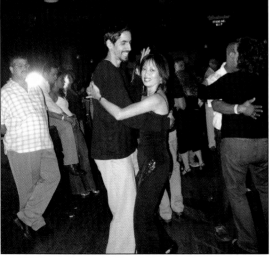

Salsa Basics

SALSA IS BEST known for its loose arm stylings, quick movements, and sensual Latin motion. Though there are two main types of salsa (ballroom and freestyle) and dozens of variations, each one, at its most fundamental level, contains the same basic steps. Salsa, when taught ballroom style, is very structured and specific. When taught freestyle, salsa is very loose, fun, and improvisational. Here, you'll learn a combination of the two so you'll be able to apply them anywhere at any time. The basic steps of both types of salsa are comprised of two sets of the quick-quick, slow rhythm.

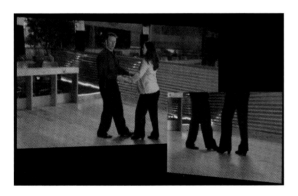

All material that you'll learn in this chapter can easily be adapted to one of the two styles. The lead-and-follow portion will be identical, but the overall look and feel of the dance will change as mentioned previously. Leaders, we'll emphasize the leads that accompany each move, regardless of the style, so both you and your partner can get the most out of the chapter.

As mentioned earlier in the chapter, the salsa is danced to 4/4 timing music, which means there are plenty of songs to practice to if you're just turning on your radio or pulling out your CD or MP3 collection. For specific songs or up-to-date playlists, it might be best to do a search online for "salsa music." You'll be sure to find a plethora of music with which to practice. You should familiarize yourself with the salsa beat and with the timing in order to recognize the dance when the opportunity arises. Before we begin the salsa, let's quickly mention our two most important rules:

1. Ladies are always right! Ladies, put your weight on your left foot so you can be ready to start with your right. (This is what's called your *ready position.*)

2. Guys always get what's left. Guys, put your weight on your right foot so you can be ready to start with your left. (This is what's called your *ready position.*)

The Eight-Count Basic

Salsa uses a quick-quick, slow rhythm in which the slows are typically considered balance steps that stabilize each partner prior to the next move. The eight-count basic of salsa is made up of two sets of rock-steps and slows. (It can also be taught as two sets of triple-steps.) Essentially, it's called out, "One, two, three (hold the count four), five, six, seven (hold the count eight)." The rock-steps are on the counts 1, 2, and again on 5, 6, just like in cha-cha.

The dance starts with the leaders rocking forward and the followers rocking back on count 1. Count 2 lets both partners finish the rock-step portion and put their weight onto the original foot. Count 3 typically comes back to your center point and allows you to stabilize. These three counts can also be said as quick-quick-slow or tri-ple-step. You're now through with half of the basic. The other half is the exact opposite, with each partner rocking with the alternate foot in the opposite direction from the first half of the basic.

On count 5, leaders will now rock back while the followers are rocking forward, and on 6 both partners will replace their weight and finish the rock-step. Count 7 is the same as 3, just with the opposite foot because it will allow you to replace your weight and hold the last count to end the basic.

Salsa, in layman's terms, is said out loud like this:

Rock-step, step, rock-step, step,

Rock-step, step, rock-step, step

If you're more mathematically inclined and like to use numbers for your steps, it's counted like this:

One, two, three . . . five, six, seven . . .

One, two, three . . . five, six, seven . . .

Salsa also incorporates what's called *Latin motion*, or *Cuban motion*, just like the cha-cha. Because the styling for the salsa is sensual and exciting, it's easy to picture what this motion should look like. For the right look and feel of Latin motion, you must use your knees rather than your hips, but again, it's not easy. Latin motion is a direct result of bending one knee slightly while the other straightens, and then vice versa. This means that when you step, you'll use the ball of your foot first, then your heel, almost as if you're digging into the ground.

Turn your toes in slightly to keep your knees from separating too much and to give the impression that your knees are working together rather than just opening up. Try to keep the space between your knees minimal while you practice your basics, and you'll be well on your way to achieving the right look and feel for your salsa.

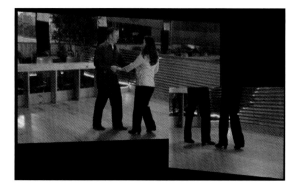

Basics in Place

To do the salsa basics in place (you can stand next to one another for this one), assume foot position 1 and be in your respective ready positions. Each of you will take three consecutive steps in place on the first three counts (in other words, step, step, step). Make sure you change weight each time. The three steps will be called out quick-quick, slow, where the slow is the one that will take up counts 3 and 4. Then, to do counts 5 through 8, you'll take three more steps and call it quick-quick, slow again. Doing the steps in place will allow you to build your rhythmic skills and understand the timing.

Another great way to practice the timing and rhythm is to clap instead of stepping. You can do this sitting down or standing because it only involves your hands. You would count the numbers 1–8 aloud and you'd clap on 1, 2, 3, and then on 5, 6, 7 each time. This is the same as quick-quick, slow, quick-quick, slow, and so on....

Next, we'll add in some motion here rather than just stepping in place. You'll want to simply rock on count 1 (changing weight), then step down on count 2 (again changing weight, but make sure your foot stays in place for the second step). Guys, you'll be rocking forward, and ladies will be rocking backwards. (Remember, your steps are opposite.) Then, you'll both do the slow step in place (and you'll hold the next count and do nothing).

Then, you'll do a rock-step the other direction (if you rocked forward first, now you'll rock back, and vice versa). Upon completion of the rock-step, you'll finish with your final slow, right back where you started, and you'll hold the last count. This same pattern will now take you through the eight-count basic, so once you've done it once, go ahead and repeat it over and over just for fun. Doing this a few times should get you familiar with the timing and the changing of weight. At the end of every eight counts, you should be ready to start back over on count 1 with your first rock-step. And yes, at the end of each basic (when you're doing them in place), you'll be in your ready position (or very close to it).

Removing the Rock

Though you've incorporated the rock-step into your basics of salsa, you'll now remove the up and down rocking portion of it, yet your footwork will remain the same. Imagine, if you will, doing the same rock-steps that you just did a moment ago, except this time, your upper torso is hardly moving at all and your feet are doing all the work. It would almost appear as though your feet are moving forward and backward without your body. Now, rather than just imagining it, give it a try. You'll notice that you can't take as big of a step and that you'll probably have to flex (or bend) your knees a little in order to step. Leaders, you'll still start with your left foot going forward and followers, you'll start with your right foot going back. The fact that your upper torso isn't moving as much now will probably make you feel a bit more restricted on the whole, but more free with your lower body. This will give you more freedom to work on your Latin motion.

A fun way to practice this is to be right next to one another and for the follower to start four counts behind the leader. (This puts you both on the same foot at the same time.) Leaders, try to mimic the size steps of your partner once she starts, because this is what you'll have to do anyway as soon as you get into the closed dance position.

Mirroring: Basics

You should now be much more comfortable with the basics in place and next to each other, so this time we'll add in a new element. For the first time, you'll now be able to see and work on the basics directly in front of your partner with everything except for the upper body. For learning your individual steps the first time, stand directly in front of each other (slightly offset). Try facing each other, as shown in the figure below, but be about two to five feet away from your partner in a mirrored position. It often helps if you're able to see the opposite steps, if for no other reason than just to validate your own. The individual steps and counts are broken down in the following list. Go through each one and make sure you're set up the way you need to be and that your steps are correct.

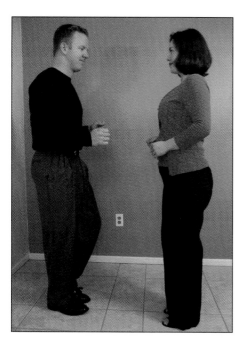

1. (Step 1 - Count 1) From a ready position, leaders will rock forward with their left foot (fourth foot position), and followers will rock back with their right foot (also in fourth foot position), with each partner changing weight to the foot that was moving by the end of step or count 1.

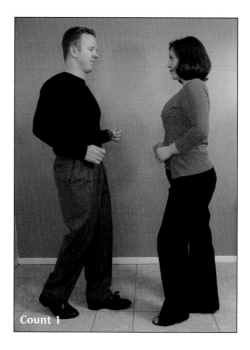

Count 1

Remember, the rock here does not include the upper torso. Also, if either partner takes too large of a step back or forward in their rock-step, it will throw you off beat and you might end up stepping on your partner.

2. (Step 2 - Count 2) Leaders, shift your weight onto your right foot (it should not have moved) as you complete the "step" portion of the rock-step (fourth foot position). Followers, shift your weight to your left foot (it should not have moved either) as you complete the "step" portion of the rock-step (fourth foot position).

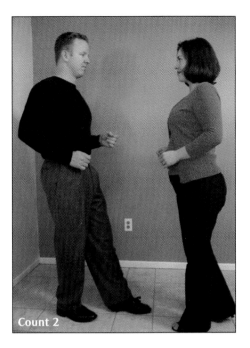

Count 2

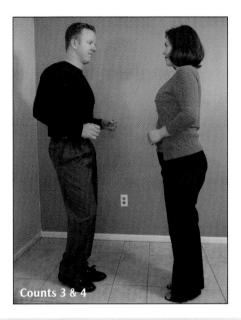

Counts 3 & 4

3. (Step 3 - Counts 3, 4) Leaders, bring your left foot back to your starting point and into the first foot position on count 3. Your weight should be firmly on your left foot with your right foot ready to step next. Followers, bring your right foot forward to your starting point, also into the first foot position on count 3. Your weight should be firmly on your right foot with your left foot ready to step next. Because this step is a slow, you'll both hold the count 4 and not step again until 5.

4. (Step 4 - Count 5) Leaders, you're now on your left foot and ready to step with your right. Your right foot will now rock backwards into the fourth foot position. Followers, you're now on your right and ready to step with your left. Your left foot will now rock forward into the fourth foot position.

As you both take Step 4 (Count 5), make sure to change your weight to the foot that is moving, but don't shift your body weight all the way over the step. Remember, your feet will step slightly beyond what your upper body will do here.

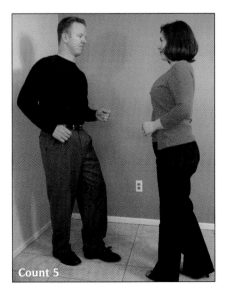

Count 5

5. (Step 5 - Count 6) Leaders, shift your weight onto your left foot (it should not have moved) as you complete the "step" portion of the rock-step (fourth foot position). Followers, shift your weight to your right foot (it should not have moved either) as you complete the "step" portion of the rock-step (fourth foot position).

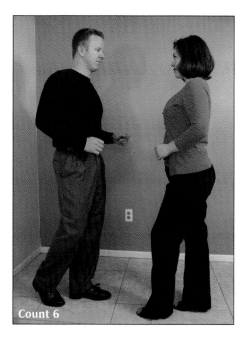

Count 6

6. (Steps 6 - Counts 7, 8) This is the opposite of Step 3. Leaders, bring your right foot forward to your starting point and into the first foot position on count 7. Your weight should be firmly on your right foot with your left foot ready to step next (your ready position). Followers, bring your left foot back to your starting point, also into the first foot position on count 7. Your weight should be firmly on your left foot with your right foot ready to step next (your ready position). Because this step is a slow, you'll both hold count 8 and not step again until 1, which is when you'd start back over.

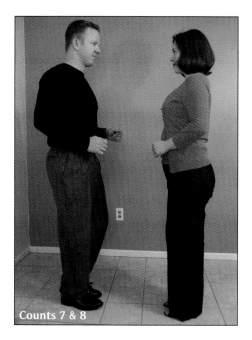

Counts 7 & 8

As you do the salsa basics footwork, be sure to keep your rock-steps under control, your steps fairly small, and your upper body fairly motionless. If it's working well, you can attempt to add Latin motion into the steps, but tread lightly. Focus on the basics first, then worry about the Latin motion; otherwise, you'll be all over the place with your hips and knees and you'll never really get the basics.

Leaders, count out loud to give the follower a chance to match you step for step when you start. The leader should say "Ready, go" or "Ready, and" on counts 5 and 7 (the equivalent of slow, slow) just prior to starting. The 5 and 7 here refer to the music that you're listening to as you prepare to take your first step. Think back to the old dance movies or stage shows in which they gave a count-down of "5-6-7-8" before starting.

As always, if either of you gets on the "wrong foot" during the exercise, just stop, laugh, and start up again after the leader counts down... "Ready, and," and you're dancing again.

Practice until you're both comfortable with the steps and the answers to each of the following questions:

- ► At the end of each basic, should you be in your ready position or in second foot position?

- ► Are there any steps that you'll take in an eight-count basic that do not include a change of weight?

- ► How many steps are taken in the eight-count basic?

- ► What are the foot positions typically used for the rock-steps in salsa?

The Eight-Count Basic as a Couple

If you've gone through the first couple of pages on the basics, you should be more than ready to dance with someone other than yourself. As such, it's time to put your upper body into the game and not just let your feet have all the fun. If you've practiced the basics enough on your own, you'll be able to focus on just the new material that's about to be introduced. Leaders, this is especially important for you because you don't want to be learning to lead at the same time as you're learning your steps.

If you skipped right to this section and didn't practice the dance on your own, you might have a tough time figuring out where any problems are if they arise. Practicing before coming together is a critical building block; the confidence each partner brings makes it much easier because you'll both have high expectations. As repeated throughout this book, social dancing is close to 25-percent skill and 75-percent attitude, so don't forget to pay attention to how you're handling situations on your own and also with your partner.

Your toolkit for the salsa basics includes:

- ► Foot position 1 (ready position, and on the counts 3 and 7 of the basic)

- ► Foot position 2 (sometimes on the counts 3 and 7 if you don't bring your feet close enough)

- ► Foot position 4 (counts 1, 2, 5, 6 of the basic)

- ► Connection point 1 (two-hand hold will be used here in the basic)

- ► Eight-count basic (essential for the salsa to work)

Position yourself so your hands (connection point 1) are engaged, and let's start the salsa. Now that you're set up, your feet are offset, and you're in your ready position, let's give it a shot. Here we go! Leaders, go ahead and give your starting count of "Ready, and," then rock forward and back, then do your step in place (the slow), then rock back and forward and finish with your final slow. Now that you got through one basic, just repeat it over and over. Is it working? You're now doing the basics of salsa...rock-step, step, rock-step, (and again!) quick-quick, slow, quick-quick, slow.... Muy bueno!

Are you feeling good about the basics yet? How do you feel about your progress with the dance thus far? If you're feeling good about the footwork and timing, it's time to turn your attention to the lead-and-follow portions. This way, we'll ensure that

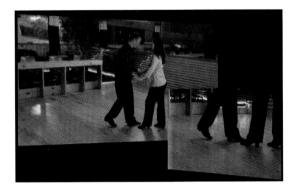

both of you understand what all is happening and how it's all broken down. Just as there's a lot to put together in other dances to make them work, salsa is no different. In fact, there's a new element to the basics in that you won't be using all four connection points to get started.

Just after the section on your new starting points will be the complete breakdown of the basics of salsa. Much like salsa, the basic can be broken into two logical pieces, each consisting of its own unique lead-and-follow aspects. Once you understand these pieces from the "basic" perspective, you'll be able to apply them to every move you do, so make sure you spend the time going through each one.

New Starting Point (Handlebars)

Rather than being in the traditional closed dance position, it's easiest if you start your salsa in a two-hand hold. (Remember this from Chapter 2?) The hand position you'll start with here most resembles handlebars because the lady's hands will be wrapped around the thumbs of the leader (see the figure at the upper-right). Leaders, open your hands up so that your fingers are pointing toward the ceiling and your thumbs are pointing toward one another. Followers, go ahead and wrap your fingers around each thumb as though they were handlebars.

Ladies, it's important that you don't squeeze because this will both hinder your ability to follow due to the amount of pressure you're providing and greatly annoy the leader because his thumbs will start tingling due to a lack of blood. Leaders, you'll now wrap your fingers around the outside and on the tops of her hands. You'll gently provide pressure just to let her know you're there and in control, but you will not squeeze or try to crush her hands. The height of the hands in this hold should be somewhere close to the follower's center point of gravity, which is near the base of the sternum. The figures below show the two-hand handlebar hold.

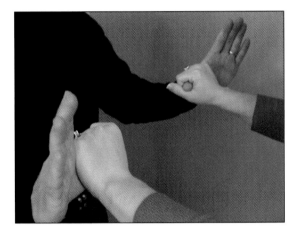

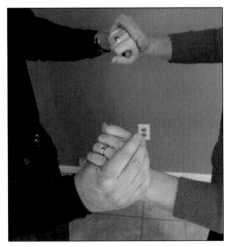

When you've mastered the handlebar hold, or one that you're both pleased with, go ahead and move into the next section. You'll quickly see how each of these parts works together to equal the sum.

Part 1

Leaders, to start your dance without any problems, you'll want to start leaning toward your partner just before you begin. Keep your right hand fairly still, but start moving your left hand toward your partner because this will cause the right side of her body to go into motion. This lean will occur somewhere around counts 7 or 8 of the "5-6-7-8" countdown prior to starting. This will allow the follower a chance to be ready by the time you're ready to start.

Followers, it's essential to have your hands fairly well connected in order to feel the leader's body heading your direction. If the leader leads this correctly, your left side shouldn't move much at all as he guides the right side of your body into the first rock-step.

Leaders, think of the rock-step here as a temporary elastic episode in which, for a brief moment, you'll be sending your partner away from you, then bringing her right back to the center point. Your left hand will be in charge and will lead her back on the first count (quick). On the second count (the second quick), your hands will stabilize, and your right hand will help put your partner onto her left foot. On the third count (the slow), your left hand will quickly take over and bring her back to center.

> **The key to making Part 1 successful is for the leader's left hand to be in motion while the right hand remains stable and ensures that the follower doesn't slip away.**

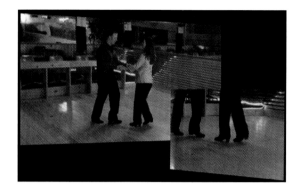

Part 2

Leaders, Part 2 of the basic is very similar to Part 1, except it reverses what was done. For the leaders, instead of rocking forward and then back, you'll now be rocking back and then forward (and it'll be with your right foot). Followers, as you know, as he rocks back with his right, this means you'll rock forward with your left.

Leaders, again, think of the rock-step here as a temporary elastic episode in which, this time, you'll be bringing your partner toward you as you step back, and then guiding her back to her center point. Your right hand will be in charge and will bring her forward (this means to pull ever so slightly) on count 5 (quick). On count 6 (the second quick on the back side), your hands will stabilize, and your left hand will help put your partner onto her right foot. On count 7 (the slow), your right hand will quickly take over and guide her back to center.

> **The key to making Part 2 successful is for the leader's right hand to be in motion while the left hand remains stable and ensures that the follower doesn't go anywhere.**

Let's practice the two main parts of the basic for a moment. Again, once you understand the dynamics of each of these pieces, you'll be able to use them in additional moves; it won't be just for the basics. Your goal for now is to get through the basics and make them look and feel natural. Guys, the more you understand how to manipulate the woman's momentum and motion through nonverbal leads, the better off you'll be. Ladies, the more you know about what feels right and why, the better you'll be at following because you'll know how to compensate when needed and you'll know when to just sit back and enjoy the dance.

Go ahead and dance through the salsa basics a few times until you're totally feeling it and understanding how it all works together. Check your progress and think through each of the pieces by going through the following list. Did you feel like any of what's in the list? We'll be adding on here in a moment, so make sure you're up and ready for it.

- ▶ **You successfully completed all eight counts (each time).**
- ▶ **You felt overwhelmed at first, but now you're feeling good about the basics.**
- ▶ **You managed to stay directly in front of your partner (slightly offset).**
- ▶ **You felt like the Latin motion wasn't quite there, but you're optimistic about it.**
- ▶ **You were smiling or caused your partner to smile with your perplexed look.**

In finalizing the salsa basics, there's no doubt that there are several types of leads going on. Just like in every other dance, the follower should feel as though her body is completely controlled by the leader. There should be enough of a lead that the follower could literally do the steps blindfolded.

Practicing with the follower blindfolded (or with her eyes closed) is a great way to practice and to test the leader's command of the dance as well as the follower's reception. The follower being blindfolded should have no impact on the couple's success on the dance floor. She should be able to do every step without using her eyes. This practicing tool works for any of the couples dances.

There's no doubt that the more time you spend on the basics, the better off you'll be. If there's a part you don't understand or one that simply isn't working, you might want to contact a local professional to get it worked out. Success is marked when everything is working together and both partners are moving effortlessly with one another.

Once you're able to do the basics without problems, you'll be ready to put it all together. (See the next page.) We'll add in a number of fun variations for you to work further with the quick-quick, slow rhythm. See whether you can follow along as we go—this is where your thinking skills will come into play. Have fun!

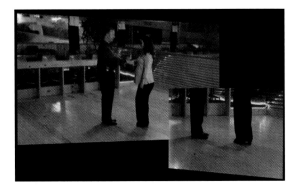

Fun Drills to Put It All Together

ONCE AGAIN, we've put together a number of fun drills and exercises for you to go through to expand your salsa knowledge while reinforcing the key elements. Instead of just picturing yourself dancing salsa, it's time to put it all together and add on. Go through each drill as they focus on different moves, leads, and thinking patterns. Soon, you'll be dancing salsa anywhere and everywhere, just for fun.

Drill 1: Shadow Dancing

Set up in your ready position with your hands extended as though your partner is connected, but do the basics on your own. Have your partner do theirs as well, just not with you because they'll be a couple of feet away. Turn some music on and dance through the basics repetitively. See who can last the longest without messing up, stopping, or getting off beat.

Drill 2: The Tortoise and the Hare

Set up in your ready position, but this time with your partner, and test several different speeds of the salsa. No music is necessary, but it can certainly help. Practice slow, normal speed (normal is what you feel most comfortable with), and then as fast as you can handle. Test your limits.

Drill 3: Side Basics

Rather than doing the basics with rock-steps back and forward, you're now going try them to the side. The basics are still elastic and you'll still come back to center; the only thing that changes is the direction of the rocks. Leaders, as soon as you're finished with a complete basic (you're standing on your right foot and the follower is on her left), you'll rock off to your left into the second foot position (still facing your partner). Then, you'll do your step in place with your right foot, then bring your left back to center on the slow. It can be called side, in place, together, then side, in place, together off to the other side with the rock-step on counts 1, 2, and on 5, 6. (Again, the rock-step is to the side instead of forward or backward.)

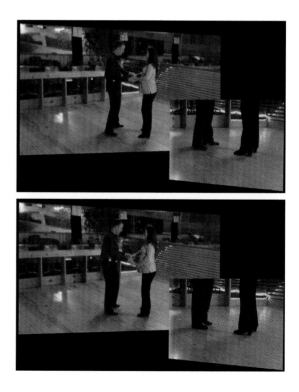

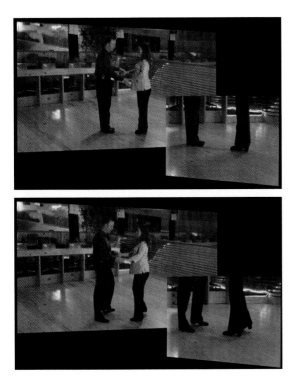

Leaders, to get the follower to move to your left, take your left hand and move it laterally to the left (while your right hand stays in place) as you step to your left. Then, bring it back to center on the slow (the step where you bring your feet together between each rock-step). To go to the right, leaders, you'll keep your left hand in place and move your right hand out while you're rocking to the right. The hands should only go out about six inches or so to provide enough of a lead for each one. Try to incorporate the side basics in with the basics you've already learned. Leaders, try to add these in every couple of basics as you're practicing. A couple of basics, then a couple of side basics, then a basic, then a side basic, and so on.

Drill 4: Two Is Better Than One

As an add-on to Drill 3 (while bouncing between the basics and the side basics), leaders can go from a two-hand hold to a one-hand hold. When practicing the basics, leaders, drop one of your two hands out of the equation and continue the basics. You might even need to change your hand from a handlebar hold to one in which the follower's hand is just placed inside of yours and your thumb is on top. Think about how you'll compensate for the other hand not being there. Go through the regular basics, and then try it with the side basics.

Now, try to go through the basics and side basics with the other hand. Which is easier for you? Now, mix it up and try a cross-handed one-hand hold as your right hand connects to the follower's right hand. Try the basics this way as well. Last, try it with each of your left hands. You'll find that, though it's possible to lead each of the basics this way, it's probably more difficult, and using two hands is better than using just one. Changing your hand positions and connection points certainly gives you some variations, though, and will let you play with the dance a bit more as you expand your salsa knowledge.

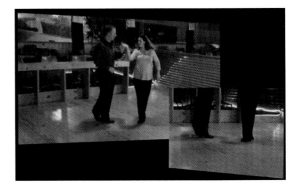

Drill 5: Underarm Turns

Here's a fun one to try. While dancing the basics using a two-hand hold, the leader will be using his right hand for the main part of the lead. The underarm turn for the ladies takes place in four counts, or half of a regular basic. The turn will be executed on the 5, 6, 7 after a normal quick-quick, slow. Leaders, you'll be pleased to know that your footwork does *not* change during this move. Keep doing the basics all the way through.

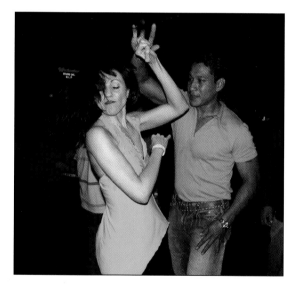

On count 5, the leader will drop his left hand (let go) and, at the same time, start raising his right hand as it's moving toward him (up and toward his face). Followers, you'll just step forward with your left foot, and you'll see and feel the hand coming up, but nothing's happened yet. On counts 6 and 7, the leader will make a "pot-stirring" motion with his right hand in a clockwise manner as he leads the follower into two separate half turns (one on count 6 and one on 7). The turns will happen together in a "step, step" manner. (In other words, there won't be a stopping point between them.) Guys, be sure to bring your hand down at the end of the turn to help stabilize your partner. Ladies, your right foot will pretty much stay in place during this entire turn because you'll use it as your center to come back to. You can try the turn on your own by stepping out with your left foot on count 5 and then turning on 6, 7. Bringing your feet back together on 7 should put you in your ready position and ready to start the basics anew.

Hot Tips for the Salsa

A S A HOT AND SENSUAL dance, the salsa has some definite styling differences that need to be pointed out. The music that accompanies the salsa helps add to the overall feel because it typically sparks the energy. Following are a number of tips, pointers, and reminders for salsa dancing now that you're feeling good about the basics and ready to move forward. Keep each one in mind as you practice your dance and prepare for your big showing.

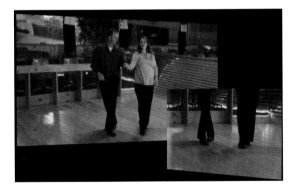

▶ **Keep your steps small and in control. The faster the music, the smaller your steps should be.**

▶ **The salsa basics are the most important. Do them well and you'll be able to do almost anything out on the social dance floor. Practice them until they become second nature.**

▶ **The eight-count basic can be danced either front and back (normal) or side to side. Either one works and has its own particular lead-and-follow elements to it.**

▶ **Soft knees are important for an overall relaxed look and to develop the starting point for your Latin or Cuban motion.**

▶ **Change weight! Whether quicks or slows, your steps should be clearly defined, should not be blended into one another, and must contain a transfer of weight.**

▶ **Minimize the amount of arm motion when it's unrelated to a lead. (This is primarily for the guys.) Too much freestyle motion will take away from the follower's ability to feel the nonverbal lead.**

▶ **Stay close to your partner. Overextending your arms during the basics will throw both of you off balance and make for a miserable time out on the dance floor.**

▶ **Keep your head up, your upper body fairly firm, and your connections intact. Strive to have a look of confidence and relaxation.**

Review and Next Steps for Your Salsa

YOU'RE MOVING right along! To wrap up the salsa, we'll do a final review to make sure you're comfortable with the major concepts and points. Go through each one and come back to this list as necessary for a quick review. Start at the beginning and work your way through each point.

Review

1. Ladies are always right! Ladies, put your weight on your left foot so you can be ready to start with your right. (In other words, get into your ready position.)

2. Guys always get what's left. Guys, put your weight on your right foot so you can be ready to start with your left. (In other words, get into your ready position.)

3. All four connection points *can* be used in the basics of the salsa (whether regular or to the side), but connection point 1 (two-hand hold) is the recommended approach.

4. The salsa basic consists of eight counts that are more important than any other step. They are:

    Rock-step (1, 2), Step (3, 4), rock-step (5, 6), step (7, 8) or Quick-quick (1, 2), slow (3, 4), quick-quick (5, 6), slow (7, 8)

5. Rock-steps are primarily done in fourth foot position. Just remember, the rock-step in salsa doesn't mean you'll rock completely over your foot. Soft knees and very little upper torso movement will help you achieve the right look.

6. The basics consist of two separate parts, and each one is led and followed a bit differently. The first part is the initial rock-step, and the second is the rock-step in the other direction. Understanding the principles behind each one of these pieces will guarantee your success with the salsa.

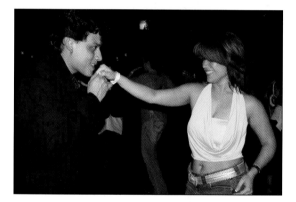

Next Steps

You're probably itching for more information regarding the salsa. At this point, you're probably ready for almost anything and everything regarding salsa. Luckily, there are many directions you can go to find more. Whether it's more about leading, following, additional moves, styling, Latin motion, or just more information on the basics, the options are plentiful. It might be best to do a search online for your particular area with the words "salsa" and your home city. See what you come up with. Ballrooms, Latin clubs, social dance clubs, community centers, and freelance instructors are all part of what you might find. It's time to get out into your community and show off your new abilities. Take it from here and see how far you can run with it. Most of all, have fun!

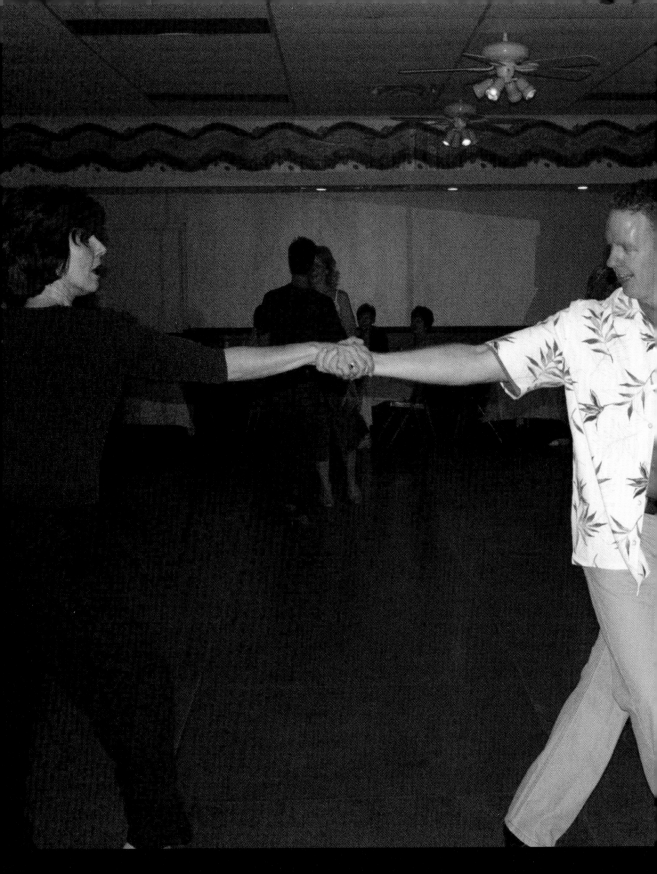

9

Picture Yourself

Doing the

Hustle

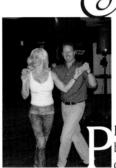

PICTURE YOURSELF doing the hustle! You might be in resplendent disco glory, complete with gold chains, polyester leisure suit, or glittery high heels. However, you might also be wearing contemporary club wear, gyrating to the beat of today's Top 40 pop hits in your local nightclub. As the leader in the hustle, you are the master of momentum and leverage. As you conquer the basic footwork and leading techniques, you will gain an appreciation for the laws of physics as you send your partner away from you and draw her back in as you rotate on the dance floor. Though you are not dancing around the dance floor, you are very conscious of your dance space—you could command the entire floor with breathtaking open moves or maintain your corner of the crowded dance floor with closed basics. The hustle allows you to take advantage of odd corners and the ever-changing topography of a freeform dance floor in a Top 40 nightclub. As the follower, fasten your safety belt and stay centered on your dance partner because you are in for the ride of your evening. Though often associated strictly with the disco music of the '70s and early '80s, the hustle is a versatile social dance that evolves with the dance music *du jour*.

The Six Ws of Hustle

THE HUSTLE IS SHROUDED by disco-ball glitter, platform shoes, blue eye shadow, and leisure suits. However, this completely American dancing phenomenon has had a much longer shelf life than some of the other artifacts of the disco era.

Who Created and Popularized the Hustle?

The hustle in its earliest form was created by the disco enthusiasts of New York City. However, the hustle was made nationally popular and tattooed its place in American pop culture through John Travolta's *Saturday Night Fever.*

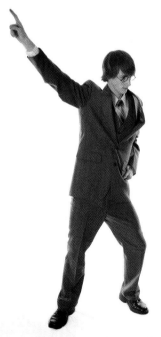

© istockphoto.com/Justin Horrocks

What Is the Hustle?

There are several different types of hustle, from line dances to the basic hustle, Latin hustle, Spanish hustle, tango hustle, four-count hustle, rope hustle, and street hustle. The dance taught in this text—and the dance done most widely today in dance studios, competitions, and nightclubs—is the three-count hustle, a derivative of the street hustle. This version of hustle is a member of the swing family and shares many attributes with the basic swing you learned earlier in this text. Like swing, hustle is danced to 4/4 time music. Also, hustle is a spot dance. Hustle is differentiated from swing in that it opens up to a slotted dance.

> A *spot dance* describes any dance in which the partners dance for the most part in one "spot" on the floor. The dance basically centers on a central point, with the partners turning, changing directions, and rotating around that point. A *slotted dance* is danced along a line, often described as railroad tracks. Generally, the follower moves forward and back along the track with the leader stepping on and off the track as he changes the follower's momentum and direction.

The dual nature of the dance is largely up to the preferences of the dancers. No matter which style is used, the follower is almost constantly spinning, and there is constant motion. The hustle is a highly adaptable dance, whether to the partner, dance floor, music, or occasion.

Where Did the Hustle Originate and Where Is It Typically Done?

As previously mentioned, the hustle was born in the nightclubs of New York City. Although not as popular as swing, the hustle has found a home at almost any event with dancing, with the exception of events where the music and dancing are exclusively Latin. Ballrooms teach a version of hustle, and you will see hustle in a Top 40 nightclub. You can also dance the hustle at a country-western nightclub! Chances are, if you turn to the Internet or just start asking around, you won't have to look long to find the haunts of local hustle enthusiasts. Just remember, you can be a hustle enthusiast without being a disco music aficionado.

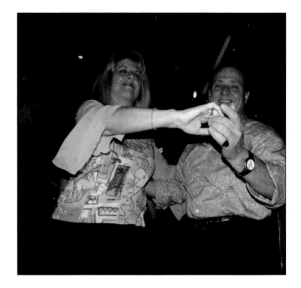

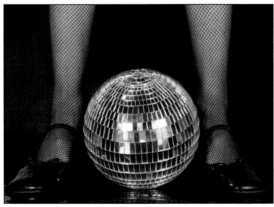

© istockphoto.com/Odelia Cohen

When Did the Hustle Become Popular and When Is the Right Time to Hustle?

The hustle was born in the early 1970s. It was a change from the dancing of the 1960s, which was predominantly solo dancing in which men and women danced together, but touching was discouraged and individuality was encouraged. The '70s ushered in the disco era. Disco enthusiasts had tired of swaying back and forth or only watching dance performers. They went to the disco dance floor and started a new phenomenon. Participation and partner dancing were in, and just watching from the sidelines was out! The first dance to emerge was the American hustle, but over the next few years many variations emerged, now almost all obsolete. The initial craze for hustle was short-lived because it was largely dependent on the popularity of *Saturday Night Fever.*

Hustle is appropriate on almost any dance floor. The right time to hustle is any time you hear appropriate music, which is 4/4 time, about 100 to 125 beats per minute, with a very smooth rhythm line. The obvious choice is disco music, but a variety of rap, techno, and Top 40 dance songs also meet this criteria. The keys are the speed of the song and the smoothness of the rhythm line.

Why Is the Hustle Danced?

Hustle is danced as a physical manifestation of the smooth, rhythmic, and energetic music by which it was inspired. For many, it is danced as a celebration of youth, as a return to their own youth, or as a representation of the cool and collected demeanor the dance requires in its full glory.

What Kind of Attire Should Be Worn?

There is no dress code for hustle dancing. The best guide is to dress for the type of event you will be attending. If you are going out to a nightclub to practice your moves, please, for your own well-being, wear club-appropriate clothing. However, if you are attending a wedding or class reunion, for the sake of those around you and your reputation, dress tastefully and in event-appropriate clothing.

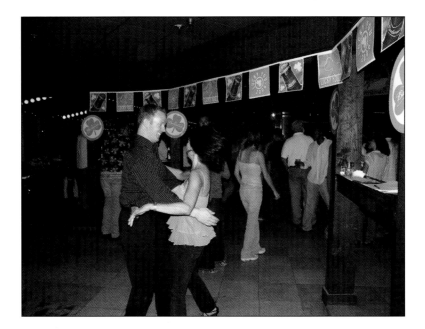

Visualize the Hustle

BEFORE STARTING the lesson plan for each dance, it's recommended you take a few minutes or so to watch the DVD that accompanies this book and view the current section. In this case, you'll be watching the hustle segment to allow your mind's eye to start processing ideas on how to get your body to do what you're watching. Visualizing the hustle will give you a good feel for what you're about to learn and will make the transition into reality that much easier.

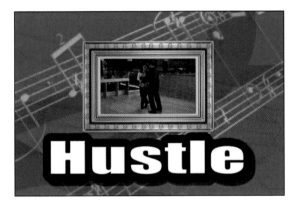

It's best if you watch the hustle section one time through without trying to do any of it. Just give your mind a chance to absorb the material so it's somewhat familiar to you when you hit replay to start the section over again. Watch how the dancers move, think about the words that are used, and picture yourself dancing the hustle.

The second time you watch the DVD, it's recommended that you take notes. Jot down the important parts of the hustle so you can engage other parts of the kinesthetic learning prior to getting up and dancing along. Write down what the connection

points are, what the basic steps are called, how many counts are in a basic, how to align with your partner, and so on. Also, write down any questions that you might have about the hustle. There's a good chance you will find the answer later in this chapter, and if it's something you're already pondering, you'll be sure to remember the answer.

You'll find that by time you get ready to stand up and try the hustle with the DVD, the dancing won't be nearly as overwhelming. Writing down the key concepts will allow you to get a jumpstart on the rest of this chapter. You'll find that after you get up and try it, you'll probably have more questions. As this chapter goes on, the steps will be broken out with screenshots from the DVD, pointers will be given on where you should be during different parts of the dance, and frequently asked questions will be addressed that should satisfy most, if not all, of your questions and then some.

The third time you view the DVD, go ahead and dance along with it. See how far you can make it just by watching and trying. You'll probably find that one of the two of you is able to pick up and understand the material more quickly than the other.

> **Just remember, everyone learns at a different pace. Be cognizant of this as you're learning with your partner. One of you might pick up certain aspects of the dance quicker than the other, and that's okay. Try to be patient and wait for the other person to grasp the material, and then move on.**

Now take a look at the rest of these pictures. All of them are taken of couples dancing the hustle. Some are formal, some are very informal, but they're all doing the same steps. See whether you can visualize yourself dancing the hustle (the dance you just watched over and over) in all these different settings. Then, picture yourself dancing the hustle at upcoming events or at local venues where you and your partner can go. Where will you go out dancing after you learn the hustle? Start thinking of the possibilities.

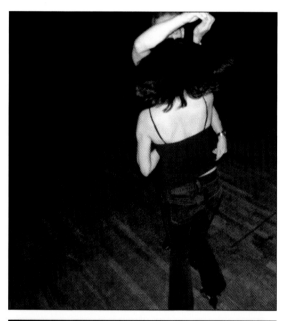

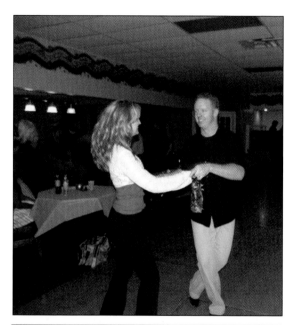

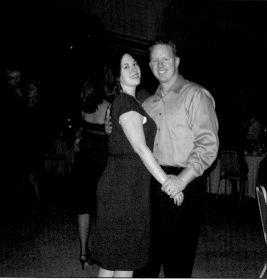

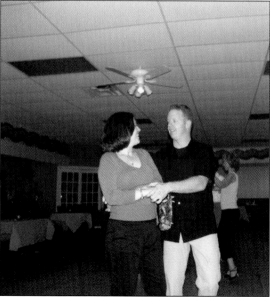

Hustle Basics

THE HUSTLE, by the nature of its background, was once considered to be the "disco" dance. Known for its smooth transitions, elastic connections, and quick circular movements on the dance floor, the hustle has transformed over the years and has grown in popularity. Now danced in many genres of music, the hustle demands a strong understanding of leading and following while portraying eye-catching moves that are fun to watch on the dance floor. The hustle is a smooth dance that offers much more than many dances due to the fact that there's constant motion.

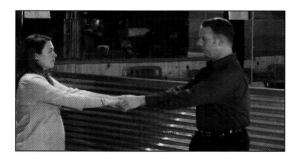

The hustle (a.k.a. the *three-count hustle*) is also sometimes called the *street hustle*, the *New York hustle*, the *rope hustle*, the *sling hustle*, the *Latin hustle*, and the *West coast hustle*. Though each is slightly different in styling, all the names refer to the same basic dance, the hustle.

As mentioned earlier in this chapter, the hustle is danced to 4/4 timing, which means there are a great number of songs to practice to, including many from your favorite disco, rap, dance, or techno CDs or MP3s. As always, it might be best to do a search online for "hustle music" or "hustle dance music" to stay current with what's playing now. At the very least, try to understand and get familiar with the timing in order to recognize the dance when the opportunity arises. You're essentially listening for a straight, constant rhythm line (think techno beats) that doesn't vary much from the beginning of the song. The best dance music for hustle should be anywhere from about 100 to 125 beats per minute.

For hustle, the same two important rules apply that you'll continue to see throughout the book:

1. Ladies are always right! Ladies, put your weight on your left foot so you can be ready to start with your right. (This is what's called your *ready position.*)

2. Guys always get what's left. Guys, put your weight on your right foot so you can be ready to start with your left. (This is what's called your *ready position.*)

The hustle basic is composed of two different timings, three counts of music, and four total steps. Don't panic—this sounds more difficult than it is. One more time on that one—two timings, three counts, and four steps. Got it? It's not as bad as it seems, though, because for the most part, the hustle is a stationary dance, although it has a lot of circular motion with it. The timing, overall, is very similar to both the two-step and the swing because the basic incorporates both slows and quicks in it, with the difference being that hustle does them in three counts, whereas two-step and swing take up six counts. The hustle basic, in layman's terms, is said out loud like this:

Quick-quick, slow, slow

If you're more mathematically inclined and like to use numbers, it's counted like this:

And-one, two, three, and-one, two, three

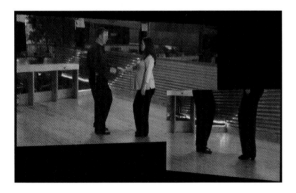

Quicks and Slows

The quicks and slows you'll do in hustle are slightly different than those in the two-step or swing. In two-step and swing, the quicks take up one whole beat apiece, and the slows take up two beats apiece. Think back for a moment and visualize yourself dancing those two dances. Remember? Now, in hustle, though you'll be doing quicks and slows, they'll be done at twice the pace.

As just stated, there are two different speeds in hustle, quicks and slows. Quicks take up a half of a beat each and slows take up one beat each.

The basic is said, "Quick-quick, slow, slow," where the "quick-quick" makes up the first beat (one-half each) and the slow, slow takes up the next two beats, which ends up being count 2 for the first slow and 3 for the second slow. For each slow you take the step on the beat, and for each quick you divide the beat in half. The first quick is on the count "and," and the second is on count 1; together, they're counted "and-1."

To summarize, following are some fun facts that you should know about the hustle:

▶ **The hustle is composed of two quicks and two slows.**

▶ **Each quick takes up only one-half of a beat.**

▶ **Each slow takes up one beat.**

▶ **A hustle basic takes up a total of three counts.**

It's also important to know that the basic for hustle should not contain any up and down motion, such as hopping or bouncing. Hustle is a smooth dance and should not look like someone is skipping or jumping rope out on the dance floor. We'll talk about this more as the chapter goes on, but it's something you should at least start thinking about.

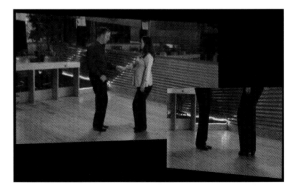

To try the hustle basics in place, assume foot position 1 and be in your respective ready positions. Next, you'll want to simply take a total of four steps in place starting with quick-quick, then doing slow, slow. Remember, the quick-quick is "and-1," and the first slow is "2," then the second slow is "3." Make sure to change weight each time and count the steps aloud. Doing the basics several times in place should get you familiar with the timing and the changing of weight.

> **This is the first time you've started a dance on a count other than 1. The "and" count essentially splits a given beat into two sections and brings a syncopated rhythm to it. You can practice this by clapping along in a repetitive three-count pattern. You'll clap on the same beats you'll be stepping on: And-one, two, three, and-one, two, three, and-one, two, three, and so on.**

After dancing and clapping the basics, you should be a bit more familiar with the timing. At the end of every three counts, you should be back in your ready position and ready to step right back down on the count "and" to start your quicks again.

> **It's recommended you practice the quicks and slows in place for at least five to ten minutes before trying them with the full moving footwork. This will allow the hustle rhythm a chance to become natural for your body. This is key because the hustle rhythm doesn't line up with the rhythm line of the music every measure. You will be completing four basics for every three measures of music.**

Mirroring

When you're comfortable with the basics in place, go ahead and move into the next steps, which will allow you to do the basics of the hustle without worrying about anything but the footwork. For learning your individual steps the first time, stand directly in front of each other. Try facing each other, about two to five feet away from your partner in a mirrored position. It's important in the hustle to see the opposite steps because both parties need to understand what their partner is doing.

1. (Step 1 - Count "and") From a ready position, leaders will do a small rock (part of a rock-step) back with their left foot (fifth foot position) and followers will rock (also part of a rock-step) back with their right foot (fifth foot position), with each partner changing weight to the foot that was moving by the end of step or count "and."

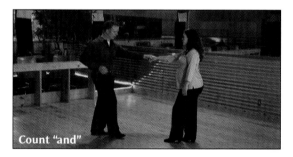

Count "and"

2. (Step 2 - Count 1) Leaders will now change their weight forward and step onto their right foot (still in fifth foot position) as they complete the rock-step. Followers will step forward onto their left foot (fifth foot position and completing the rock-step). Each partner will change weight to the foot that was moving by the end of step or count 1.

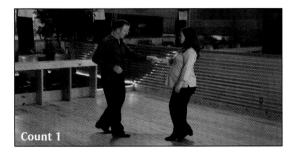

Count 1

3. (Step 3 - Count 2) Leaders will now step left into a second foot position with their left foot, and followers will step right with their right foot (also into a second foot position). Although you're stepping into foot position two, make sure the steps are small and controlled. Hustle, as quick as it is, won't allow for large steps because you won't have the time to complete them. Make sure you change weight to the foot that was moving (in other words, no tap-steps).

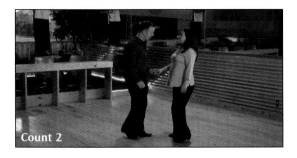

Count 2

4. (Step 4 - Count 3) Leaders will now step right into a second foot position with their right foot, and followers will step left with their left foot (also into a second foot position). Although you're stepping into foot position two, make sure the steps are small and controlled (just like in Step 3). Step 4 (the one you're learning now) is really nothing more than just stepping in place, though you have to change your weight. Leaders, when it says to step right with your right foot, this means you'll essentially just put your weight straight down onto your right foot because it's already in position after your left foot moved off into the second foot position. Followers, the same applies to your step on this one: Just do the steps in place.

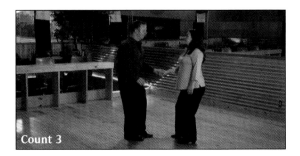

Count 3

There is no hopping in hustle! When doing the rock-step, try not to have any up and down motion. Observers should not be able to see your head go up and down during this dance.

Hopefully you already did several miles of two-step and hours and hours worth of swing before ever trying this one. If so, you're already comfortable with the quicks and slows that you're working on now. The steps are similar in hustle, but you still need some practice so they become ingrained in your muscle memory. Try dancing the steps over and over right there in front of your partner and counting them aloud. Leaders, this is your role, and you should give the verbal starting points such as "Ready, and," "Ready, go," or "5-6-7-8," or something to that effect to get you both going.

> **If either partner gets on the "wrong foot" during the exercise, just stop, laugh, and start up again after the leader counts it off . . . "5-6-7-8," and you're back dancing again.**

Practice the hustle until you're both comfortable with the steps and the answers to each of the following questions:

▶ **What foot position should I be in while doing the quicks?**

▶ **How many steps do I take during the three-count basic?**

▶ **How many counts (beats) does each slow take up?**

▶ **How many counts (beats) does each quick take up?**

The Hustle Basic as a Couple

NOW THAT YOU'RE both experts on doing the basics on your own, it's now time to try them together as a couple. Are you sure you're ready and that your feet can do the quick-quick, slow, slow once your upper body is engaged? If you skipped right to the dancing and didn't practice it on your own, you might have a tough time figuring out where any problems are if they arise. Practicing before coming together is critical to the success of each partner, and it's easier if you come in with steps that are closer to being set in stone with your body. As continuously mentioned, social dancing is not all skill; in fact, it's probably closer to only about 25-percent skill with the remainder being your attitude. If you're genuinely excited and ready to practice and learn, chances are you'll have no problem figuring out where things might have gone wrong with the steps you encounter. That said, you'll be all set for a great time out on the floor.

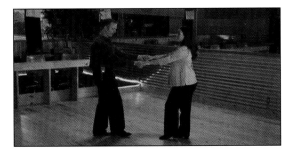

Your toolkit for the hustle basics includes:

▶ **Foot position 1 (Ready position to start and at any time during the dance when you have to start over.)**

▶ **Promenade dance position (Refer to Chapter 2 if you need a refresher!)**

▶ **Foot position 3 (the rock-step portion of the basics while in closed/promenade dance position)**

▶ **Connection points 1–4 (All will be used in the closed and promenade dance position basics; the hold will be similar to that in the swing, with the leader's left hand down closer to the waistline. Connection point 1 will be used by itself as a one-hand hold in the majority of the open figures in the basics of hustle.)**

▶ **Three-count basic (Remember: a total of four steps in the basic.)**

Are you ready to start hustling with your partner? I'm not sure whether "hustling" is the right term, but it's fun to say in this situation and it fits, so we'll go with it. Let's give it a shot.

First, you'll want to get into your closed dance position (opened slightly into the promenade position) with your partner (use all four connection points) and be in your ready position. Also, you'll want to make sure you're slightly offset so no one gets stepped on. Leaders, go ahead and give your countdown (5-6-7-8 or however you choose) and start out with your left rock-step, and then replace your weight on your right foot (quick-quick or "and-1"), then slow it down a bit and do your first slow (only one count) and then do your second one in place.

Now, start it over again and do all four of the steps back to back to back to back...quick-quick, slow, slow. And now, just repeat it over and over. Excellent—you're doing the hustle! Keep going and see how far you both can make it. It will feel a bit awkward just doing these steps over and over in place, but it'll help give you the foundation you'll need to get into the next part. Don't rush through the basics just to get to the turns. Without the basics, none of the rest of it will make sense.

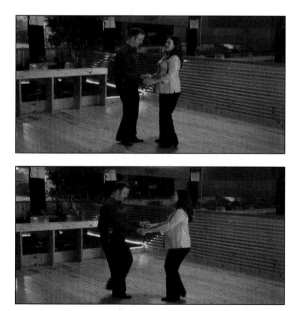

As it happens with each basic, you now must turn your attention to making this a lead-and-follow dance. Get back to your ready position and let's make sure the leaders are actually leading this one and the followers are following it. Leaders, just like

in any dance, you have four connection points that you will use here to help you. The two most important ones for both partners are connection points 1 and 2. Leaders, your upper body must be in synch with your lower body on this one because you'll need the ability to swiftly (yet gently) move your partner around. If your upper and lower body fall out of synch, you will send mixed messages to your partner and quickly fall off beat.

Leaders, your arms should not be pushing or pulling; rather, they should be acting like springs. The controlled movements of your hands and arms should work together to create a spring-like feeling, yet neither partner should feel as if his or her arm is being ripped from its socket. The leads in hustle are a primary result of physics, leverage, and timing, rather than of strength or sheer force.

Did it work? If so, you did each of the following (you should aim for at least four of the five):

- ▶ **You successfully completed the three-count basic (all four steps).**
- ▶ **You both changed weight four times during the basic.**
- ▶ **You managed to stay directly in front of each other (slightly offset).**
- ▶ **You both had a smile on your face or caused your partner to smile.**
- ▶ **You both managed to get through the basics without hopping.**

Leaders, we continue to emphasize the following point: If you give a lady a choice (on the dance floor), she'll take it! If you leave the door open for interpretation, you never know what you'll end up with. Nothing personal here, ladies—it would be the same if you were leading.

Okay, leaders, take your partner in closed dance position slightly offset (all four connection points) and try the basics again. Practice the basics from a starting point over and over until you're comfortable with starting directly into the quick, quick. Then, have your follower close her eyes and see whether she can follow what you're doing and when you're starting. Leaders, prior to starting the quick-quick (on the "Ready, and" part), it helps if you lean slightly to your left and then back to your right (like a small sway) to allow the follower's body to start moving. This movement will place her weight firmly on her left foot while her momentum sets her up for an easy rock-step. If the lead is correct, your partner will match you step for step and also in the speed. If the follower is having difficulty (other than not understanding the basics), there's a better than 90-percent chance it has something to do with the lead.

Rock-Steps

It's very important in the hustle to take small steps, especially during the rock-steps. It's equally as important that you don't step down onto the entire foot during the rock-step, or else you might never be able to recover the timing that you might lose because you only have half a beat to work with. When doing the rock-step in the hustle basics, it's best to think of it as pushing off as you compress into the ground the area between your big toe and the ball of your foot.

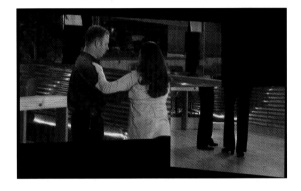

Your knees should be slightly flexed during the rock-step, so the fact that you're not stepping all the way onto your rocking foot shouldn't make you elevate (lift up) as you did in swing or in waltz. And, though you're not stepping onto the entire foot area, there is still a change of weight that must take place.

Closed to Open Position (and Then Back to Closed)

NOW THAT YOU have a firm grasp on the basic footwork, it's time to open up your dance a bit and start the movement. Most importantly, though, before you begin, take note that regardless of how much you move around, there's no change to the timing of the quick-quick, slow, slow part of the dance. Keep that in check and you'll be fine throughout the rest of this chapter.

Going from a closed (promenade) dance position to an open position will most resemble a whip, a slingshot, or even a boomerang. The leaders will act as though they're tossing the followers out to a one-hand hold, yet it will be nothing more than a well-guided lead that allows the followers to break away. Following is a step-by-step depiction of what happens to pull this one off.

Part 1: Closed to Open

Leaders, to start this move, you'll first prepare your body. For the greatest amount of leverage, you'll always want to do your rock-step the exact opposite of where your partner is doing hers. Think of the rock-step in the hustle as a constant mirror image. When you go to lead your partner from a closed dance position to an open one, it's best to end with a side-rock, rather than in a fifth or extended fifth foot position. The side-rock (second foot position) will enable you (the leader) to rock away from your partner to create the leverage or spring-like motion that you'll need to quickly move your partner across your body and away from you.

On the "and" count (the first quick), the leaders will rock out to their left side and the followers will rock back as normal. On the 1 (the second quick), the leader will use his right hand to start bringing the follower across his body from right to left. The leader's right hand will curve in toward his chest, which will allow the follower's right shoulder to also start turning toward the inside of the partnership. (The follower's left foot should now be aimed more toward the leader because it's preparing her for her turn.)

Please note that the majority of this lead is created with the leader's right hand. In fact, this can be led without any connection between the leader's left hand and the follower's right hand. Leaders, if you find yourself using your left hand to "pull" your dance partner across your body through this part of the move, release this connection point and lead the step with your right hand alone.

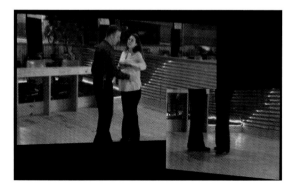

On count 2 (the first slow), the leaders will step across their right foot with their left foot as they travel to the right and turn slightly to the left. At the same time (on 2), the leaders will release their right hand as they bring the follower through, and the followers will roll out to a one-hand hold as they turn a half turn to their left. The turn to the left will be a natural fallout of the forward momentum created by the opposing rock-steps and the release of the leader's right hand (connection point 2).

On count 3 (the second slow), the leaders will square up with the followers and do a small step (pretty much in place) with their right foot to help balance out and slow down the movement. You're now in a one-hand hold, facing each other with momentum going away from one another.

Part 2: Open to Closed (the J-Lead)

At this point, both partners will do a regular rock-step (on the "and-1") of the next basic, only this time it will be in the fourth foot position (straight back). Because both partners are facing one another and the elastic look is created by both partners going opposite ways (like a rubber band), it's best to do your rock-steps in this manner. The next part is called a *J-Lead* because the leader will be making a movement with his left hand that resembles a J.

Leaders, as you step slightly left on count 2 (the first slow) with your left foot, your left hand will be traveling toward you as if it were traveling down the long "stem" portion of the J. You're essentially getting out of the way of the follower because she'll be heading directly toward you. Leaders, your hand coming in toward you will cause the follower to step forward with her right foot and start to turn slightly toward her right as you start the rounded portion of the J at the bottom.

The J-Lead will continue through count 3 (the second slow) as the J is completed by the leader pulling his hand in toward himself, slightly to the left to form the hook of the J, and slightly back away from himself to form the short end of the J. This J motion, which in execution should feel as though you were writing a giant J on a flat surface parallel to the floor, will draw the follower in toward the leader, and then turn her to squarely face the leader in a closed dance position. Leaders, between the counts 2 and 3 as the follower comes back in beside you (and while your left hand is executing the J-Lead), you'll want to place your right hand back into connection point 2. Your right hand will connect while moving off to the right with the follower's momentum. This connection point will be what the follower needs to feel secure and to slow down.

When you're fully connected again and upon completion of the J-Lead, the leaders have the option of repeating the closed-to-open portion again (which means the leaders would do the side-rock next) or doing the normal rock-step back without the leverage. It all depends on what the leader's next move is.

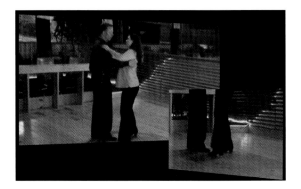

Turning Basics (Left and Right)

NOW THAT YOU have the basics down and you're able to go from a closed dance position to an open dance position and then back again, it's time to add some circular elements. Rather than just standing there in place and doing the hustle, you'll now rotate and do the basics with both left and right turns. Keep in mind that no matter which direction you're heading, you still have to maintain the basic quick-quick, slow, slow rhythm. We'll start with left turns, and then work our way to the right ones.

Leaders, the titles of the following moves are for your benefit because you're the one who has to remember and lead them. A left turn means you'll be turning to your left, and a right turn means you'll be turning to your right.

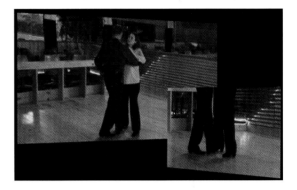

Leaders, at the same time as you're stepping out with your left foot, your right hand (connection point 2) will be leading your partner across to your left to get her to turn left with you. (Connection point 1 is also used with a little pulling motion, but it's not the primary lead on this one.) Ladies, you'll step across and in front of the leader here with your right foot on count 2 (the first slow), and you should feel balanced and ready to step with your left foot for count 3.

Left Turns

Leaders, to execute the left turns, you'll need to be in your promenade dance position, ready to step with your left foot. You'll first do a rock-step in fifth foot position as you would with the normal promenade basic. Upon completion of the rock-step, you'll take a small step out with your left foot on count 2 (the first slow) to an extended third foot position (with your left foot in front rather than your right foot, as in the rock-step).

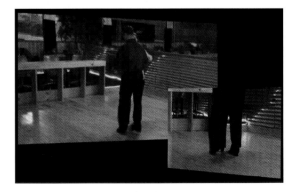

On 3 (the second slow), leaders will step slightly forward with their right foot as the followers step slightly back with their left. The leader's left hand will now come back into play because it will help stop the momentum on count 3. After 3 comes the next rock-step, which should also be led by the leader's left hand. A slight nudge (an easy push) by the leader's left hand should cause the follower to step back with her right foot into the rock-step.

Right Turns

Leaders, to execute the right turns, you just need to concentrate on turning to the right instead of the left. Because you start with your left foot and this a right turn, you'll have to wait until your right foot is free to turn. After you do your normal rock-step (fifth foot position), you'll step out with your left foot into a second foot position, yet slightly forward on 2 (almost into an extended third because your left foot will be slightly angled on this slow step). Followers, on 2 you'll be taking a small step forward with your right foot. If the leader is leading it correctly, your foot should be slightly turned to the right at the beginning of the step to help you prepare for the upcoming turn.

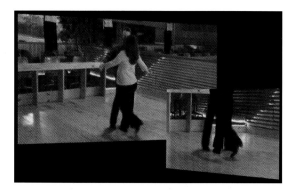

Then, leaders, on the third count (the second slow), you'll start and finish the turn by stepping with your right foot into an extended third foot position (with your right foot being the foot in the back). At the same time as you're stepping with your right foot, you'll also be turning the follower slightly to her right. (Followers, you'll be turning on your right foot and getting ready to step with your left foot) and placing her in front of you with her weight on her left foot on 3. Upon completion of count 3, the leaders have the option of doing another rock-step into a right turn, a left turn, a closed-to-open basic, or almost anything that they choose.

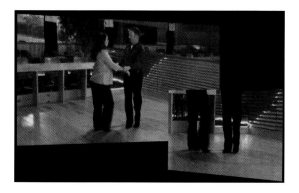

Mixing the Turns

Leaders, this is where you get to test out your new skills. Rather than just doing left turns, then stopping, then doing right turns, then stopping, or doing one every now and then, you're going to work on transitions and your lead. Get into your closed dance position and start your basics. After doing a couple of basics, try to do three left turns, one basic in place, two right turns, and then a closed-to-open-to-closed basic. What you're working on here are the dynamics of the leads of each, and both of you should work through your parts until you both nail them every time. Mix it up in any grouping you want, just as long as you're thinking through each one. Have fun with this, but take it seriously. Left and right turns are essential for a successful hustle.

Fun Drills to Put It All Together

FOLLOWING ARE a number of drills, exercises, and fun new steps set up specifically for you to practice and add to what you've learned. Try each drill as they focus on different elements, leads, and thinking patterns. By the end of these drills, you should feel confident enough to try your hustle almost anywhere.

Drill 1: Solo Dancing

Set up in your ready position in your dance frame and do the basics on your own. Have your partner do theirs as well, just not with you. Turn on some hustle music if you have it (if not, try it without) and dance through everything you just learned, including the basics, the left turns, the right turns, and the closed-to-open-to-closed positions. See who can last the longest without messing up, stopping, or getting off beat. You'll be dancing by yourself, but working on the leading, following, and footwork portions for all of the moves in your repertoire. Practicing this way will help lock the moves into your long-term memory.

Drill 2: The Tortoise and the Hare

Set up in your ready position, but this time with your partner, and test several different speeds of the hustle. No music is necessary, but it helps if you have it because you'll have fun practicing slowly, at normal speed (you'll decide what normal is), and then as fast as you can handle.

Drill 3: Open or Closed?

In this drill, you'll nearly double the amount of hustle moves that you learned just by changing your position and practicing the basics. Leaders, as you're dancing your basics, drop connection point 2, move slightly away from your partner, extend your hands to offer an open dance position, and keep the basics going. You still have to lead the basics, but now you'll do it with both of your hands in front of you.

Once you master the basics again, try the left and right turns. One thing to note in hustle is that whenever you're in an open position and you come in close to one another, your hands will slightly extend outward to maintain the same height from the ground. Then, as you separate for the rock-steps, your hands will come back to the center point. Once you get it, mix and match and go from a closed dance position to an open dance position at random times while you practice the moves.

Drill 4: Hula Dancing

Using a hula hoop is a great way to practice the leading and following for the hustle. Leaders, you're in charge as usual, and followers, you just need to set up inside the hoop with your arms around the outside and your hands wrapped back up under and on the inside of the hoop itself. Practice everything you learned in this chapter. This drill can be done with or without music.

Hot Tips for the Hustle

AS ONE OF THE BEST-recognized disco dances of all time, you should now have a good feel for what the hustle is all about. Following are a number of tips and pointers that you can go through to help reinforce what you've learned.

▶ Don't bounce! When doing the rock-steps (especially), try to keep your level the same as when you're doing the slows.

▶ Hustle is a fast-moving dance that requires both partners to keep their heads up and their eyes open. Either partner looking down detracts from the look of the dance, throws off the balance of the couple, and could easily cause accidents on the dance floor due to not paying attention.

▶ Hustle should be smooth, almost like gliding. Dancers should look as though they're effortlessly moving back and forth with their partner. Up and down (vertical) motion should not be visible as couples execute the basics.

▶ Maintaining frame and connection is critical in the hustle. The leader must be able to move in any direction at all times, and all connection points must be engaged for effective maneuverability.

▶ Stay close to your partner, but not too close! If you get too far away, your arms will feel as if they're being pulled from their sockets. If you're too close, there will be no movement at all.

▶ Be aware of your surroundings and others on the floor.

▶ The basics in the hustle are more important than anything. Spend more time practicing the quick-quick, slow, slow than anything else.

▶ The continuous flow of movement should be prevalent in the hustle. If the dance looks or even feels like it's choppy or bouncy, it probably is.

▶ Take small, manageable, controlled steps! This enables you to avoid the look of skipping, hopping, bouncing, or stutter-stepping through your basics.

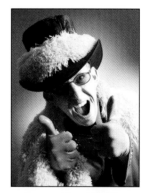

© istockphoto.com/ Joshua Blake

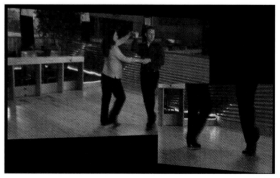

Review and Next Steps for Your Hustle

STUPENDOUS! If you're starting from the beginning, you've now completed seven dances. To ensure your comfort and to do a final recap, we're going to run back through the major points of what you've learned. Go through each one and come back to this list as necessary for a quick review. Start at the beginning and work your way through each point.

Review

1. Ladies are always right! Ladies, put your weight on your left foot so you can be ready to start with your right. (In other words, get into your ready position.)

2. Guys always get what's left. Guys, put your weight on your right foot so you can be ready to start with your left. (In other words, get into your ready position.)

3. The hustle basic consists of a total of three beats: quick (1/2), quick (1/2), slow (1), slow (1).

4. The hustle basic is counted "quick ("and")-quick ("1"), slow ("2"), slow ("3")." There are still some folks who count it starting with the slows first: "Slow ("1"), slow ("2"), quick ("and")-quick ("3")," but there's no difference in the way it's danced.

5. Rock-steps are typically done on the quick-quick portion of the dance (at least in the basics) and are done in fifth foot position when in closed/promenade dance position or in fourth foot position when in an open dance position (when you are directly opposite your partner).

6. All four connection points are used in the basics of the hustle. Connection points 1 and 2 are the most prevalent in the leads for the basics.

7. Hustle is a smooth dance and therefore should be danced at the same level (without lilt, bounce, or hopping).

8. Connection point 2 is primarily used when you are going from a closed dance position to an open one, whereas connection point 1 (with a J-Lead) is best used for going from an open to a closed dance position.

9. Left turns start with the leader stepping out to an extended third foot position with his left foot on the first slow.

10. Right turns start with the leader stepping out to an extended third foot position with his right foot on the second slow.

Next Steps

Are you comfortable and ready for more? Assuming you're now competent and confident, you'll be looking for more information on the leading and following portions of hustle and how to quickly add moves to your dance. There are not as many places where the hustle is danced, though it's becoming more prevalent at ballrooms, country nightclubs, and especially nightclubs where disco is played. A few searches on the Internet might help you find the right venue for you in your hometown. As you just found out, the hustle can be a lot of fun, and it's great exercise because you're constantly moving. Put on some funky disco threads and get out there and join the fun!

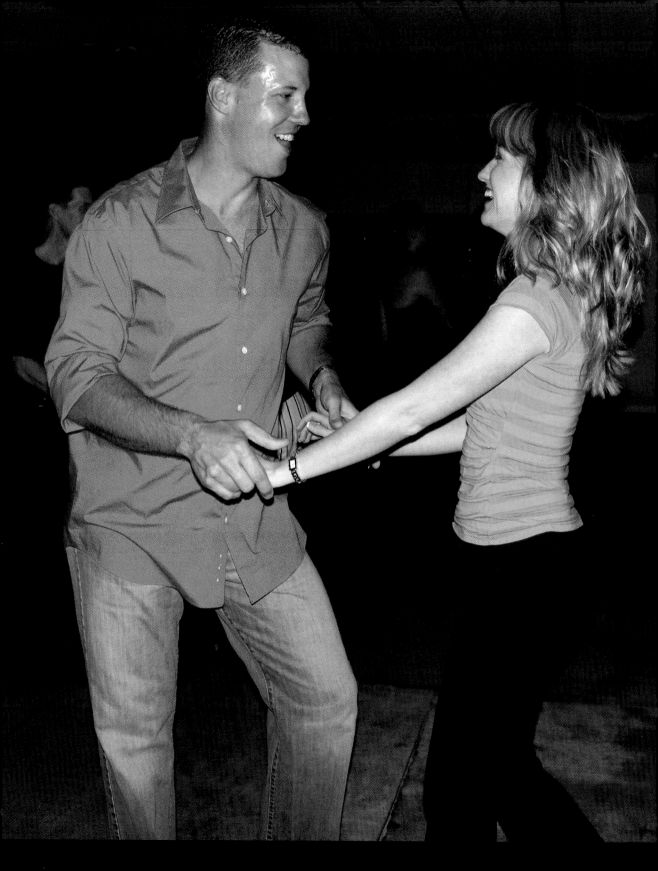

10

Picture Yourself

Dancing the West Coast Swing

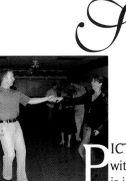

PICTURE YOURSELF on a crowded dance floor
with 50 other West coast swing enthusiasts. The air
is infused with the deep bass of the blues backbeat
that provides the under-girding for all music associated
with the West coast swing. As you look around the dance
floor you realize that your companions come from all
walks of life, but are united by a passion for the unique,
intense, partner-dance experience that West coast swing
provides. As a leader, you are in charge of the traffic pattern that you and your partner will create within your slot
on the dance floor. Though your part of the dance is not
marked by much movement of foot, it is branded by the
rapid thought patterns and intricate leading action that
make West coast swing the "dancer's dance." As a follower, you are prepared to hang onto your socks because
you will be burning up the dance floor as the showpiece
of the West coast swing. To successfully dance the West
coast, you must completely embrace the three rules of
following without restraint. You must not hold on, you
must never let go, and you must not think! The challenges
associated with the varying time in West coast, as well as
the intricate footwork, make mastery of the West coast
swing a challenge for dancers at every skill level.

The Six Ws of West Coast Swing

THE WEST COAST swing is a challenging dance that has evolved from spin-off status into a separate dance with a fervent following and a thriving competition circuit.

Who Popularized the West Coast Swing?

The West coast swing was created by the jitterbug dancers in Hollywood, California. Dean Collins as an individual was instrumental in the development of the West coast swing. He brought the Savoy-style Lindy to California and started adding his own flavor as he taught it. The other key players in the development of West coast swing were the movie producers of the 1930s and 1940s, the local dancers at nightclubs, and the soldiers and sailors

of the United States military who spread the West coast swing along with other versions of jitterbug around the world. As Arthur Murray looked to document and create curriculums for the various dances of the day, Laurie Haile documented and immortalized the swing of Dean Collins and other California dancers as Western swing, which later became known as West coast swing (in comparison to East coast swing or Eastern swing).

What Is the West Coast Swing?

West coast swing is the most intricate of the partner dances taught in this text. The basic is a six-count basic, but moves from elementary through a highly advanced range, from six to twelve or more counts per move. This is very unique to West coast swing, differentiating it even from the other swing dances. Another key attribute that differentiates West coast swing from Lindy and other versions of swing as well as most non-swing dances is the slot.

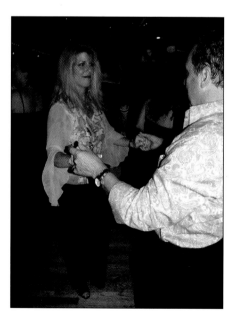

A *slotted dance* describes a dance that is danced along a line, often described as railroad tracks. The follower generally moves forward and back along the track with the leader stepping on and off the track as he changes her momentum and direction.

There are a few stories circulating regarding the reason for the slot. The first attributes the slot to Hollywood. Because the wide-angle camera lens had not been invented yet in the 1930s and 1940s, producers had the dancers line up in straight lines to create the camera shots. The dancers began dancing in slots so the camera saw their profiles for the entire dance, rather than their backs as they rotated, allowing the audience to see a lot more dancing. This became such a common practice that the slots stuck. The second story attributes the slot to the crowded dance floors of Los Angeles, which forced the dancers into slotted-type movement to avoid hitting each other. The third story attributes the slotted style of West coast swing to the practice of dancing in the aisles at big-band music concerts in the concert halls of Los Angeles. Most likely the slots evolved through the influence of all three historical factors as the West coast swing developed.

Where Did the West Coast Swing Originate and Where Is It Typically Done?

As previously mentioned, West coast swing was born in southern California. The soldiers and sailors of World War II spread the West coast swing around the country and throughout the world along with all of the other versions of swing danced during that era. Today, West coast swing can be found in every corner of this country, with a thriving competition circuit and a fervent following.

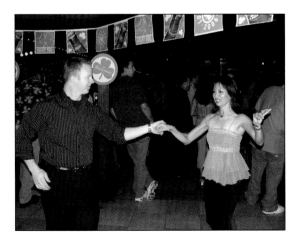

When Did the West Coast Swing Become Popular and When Is the Right Time to West Coast Swing?

West coast swing was born in the 1930s, when Dean Collins brought his version of the Savoy-style Lindy and adapted it to the cameras and dance floors of southern California. Since then, West coast swing has remained a living dance, evolving with the music selections of the day while still maintaining loyalty to the blues from which it was born.

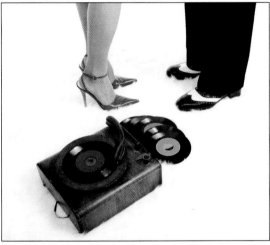

© istockphoto.com/Lisa Gagne

West coast swing is appropriate on almost any dance floor. The right time to West coast swing is anytime you hear appropriate music, which is 4/4 time, about 100 to 125 beats per minute. The obvious choice is blues music, but a variety of Top 40 dance songs also meet this criteria. The keys are the speed of the song and the swinging rhythm.

Why Is the West Coast Swing Danced?

West coast swing was born as an adaptation to physical surroundings and the evolving need for challenge to the dancers. People who love dancing and studying the art of lead and follow dance it. Because there are so many variations of West coast swing, it can be danced as a swing dance, a seductive dance, a rhythm dance, or simply as an exercise for a dancer.

What Kind of Attire Should Be Worn?

There is no dress code for West coast swing. The best guide is to dress for the type of event you will be attending. If you are going out to a nightclub to practice your moves, please, for your own well-being, wear club-appropriate clothing. However, if you are attending a wedding or class reunion, for the sake of those around you and your reputation, dress tastefully and in event-appropriate clothing.

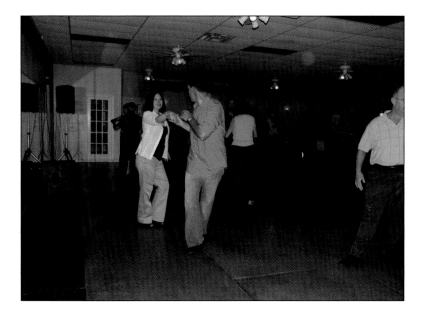

Visualize the West Coast Swing

BEFORE STARTING the lesson plan for each dance, it's recommended you take a few minutes or so to watch the DVD that accompanies this book and view the current section. In this case, you'll be watching the West coast swing (hereafter, referred to as "WCS" in this chapter) segment to allow your mind's eye to start processing ideas for how to get your body to do what you're watching. Visualizing the WCS will give you a good feel for what you're about to learn and will make the transition into reality that much easier.

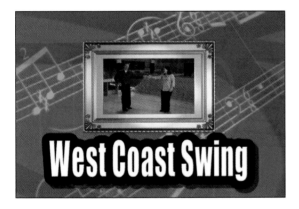

It's best if you watch the WCS section one time through without trying to do any of it. Just give your mind a chance to absorb the material so it's somewhat familiar to you when you hit replay to start the section over again. Watch how the dancers move, think about the words that are used, and picture yourself dancing the WCS.

The second time you watch the DVD, it's recommended that you take notes. Jot down the important parts of the WCS so you can engage other parts of the kinesthetic learning prior to getting up and dancing along. Write down what the connection points are, what the basic steps are called, how many counts are in a basic, how to align with your partner, and so on. Also, write down any questions that you might have about the WCS. There's a good chance you will find the answer later in this chapter, and if it's something you're already pondering, you'll be sure to remember the answer.

You'll find that by time you get ready to stand up and try the WCS with the DVD, the dancing won't be nearly as overwhelming. Writing down the key concepts will allow you to get a jumpstart on the rest of this chapter. You'll find that after you get up and try it, you'll probably have more questions. As this chapter goes on, the steps will be broken out with screenshots from the DVD, pointers will be given on where you should be during different parts of the dance, and frequently asked questions will be addressed that should satisfy most, if not all, of your questions and then some.

The third time you view the DVD, go ahead and dance along with it. See how far you can make it just by watching and trying. You'll probably find that one of the two of you is able to pick up and understand the material more quickly than the other.

Just remember, everyone learns at a different pace. Be cognizant of this as you're learning with your partner. One of you might pick up certain aspects of the dance quicker than the other, and that's okay. Try to be patient and wait for the other person to grasp the material, and then move on.

Now, take a look at the rest of these pictures. All of them are taken of couples dancing the WCS. Some are formal, some are very informal, but they're all doing the same steps. See whether you can visualize yourself dancing the WCS (the dance you just watched over and over) in all these different settings. Then, picture yourself dancing the WCS at upcoming events or at local venues where you and your partner can go. Where will you go out dancing after you learn the WCS? Did you come up with anyplace? It's very versatile, so start thinking of the possibilities....

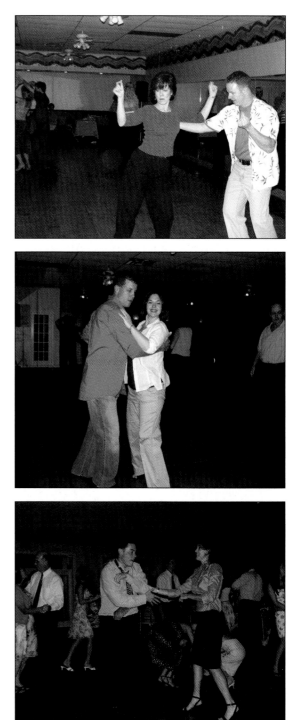

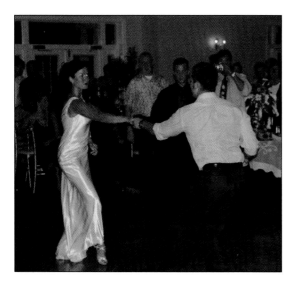

West Coast Swing Basics

W EST COAST SWING can best be described as a slotted dance with strong roots in the basics and fundamentals of lead-and-follow dance. Having said that, once you understand the basics, the world of WCS is wide open, and a dancer can go almost any direction. Styles of WCS include classic, contemporary, sophisticated, funky, retro, sexy, Latin, country, and of course, those related to the blues. WCS can be danced almost anywhere, in any dance situation, and with anyone else who understands the basics to music ranging from 100–130 beats per minute (give or take a few beats). The basics include walking-steps, tap-steps, and triple-steps (anchor-steps).

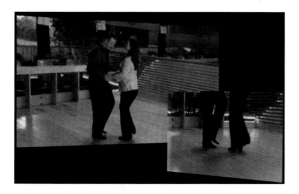

Walking-steps **include one change of weight per beat,** *tap-steps* **include one change of weight for every two beats, and** *triple-steps* **(***anchor-steps***) include three changes of weight for every two beats.**

As previously mentioned, the WCS is danced to 4/4 timing, which means the number of songs you can practice to is quite extensive, whether you're just turning on your radio or pulling out your CD or MP3 collection. For specific songs or up-to-date playlists, it might be best to do a search online for "West coast swing music" and find a few songs from whatever genre of music is your favorite, and then practice along. There's a lot to choose from! Once you hear some of the music, you'll know what to look for and you'll be able to recognize the dance when the opportunity arises. Before we begin the WCS, let's recap our two most important rules:

1. Ladies are always right! Ladies, put your weight on your left foot so you can be ready to start with your right. (This is what's called your *ready position.*)

2. Guys always get what's left. Guys, put your weight on your right foot so you can be ready to start with your left. (This is what's called your *ready position.*)

The Six-Count Basic

The six-count slotted basic of West coast swing is made up of two walking-steps, a tap-step, and a triple-step (an anchor-step). The term "slotted" is used because the dancers dance on an imaginary line and travel back and forth on it, as opposed to a circular or progressive dance, in which the dancers move around the dance floor. Picture the slot as something similar to a train track that you'd be dancing within. Luckily, the follower does the majority of the movement in this dance. That's right, guys: You get to dance in place for this one! (That doesn't mean your feet don't move, though.)

To give you a mental image of the dance, WCS starts out with the leaders and followers standing a couple of feet apart, facing each other, and typically connected by a one-hand hold. The leader draws the follower toward himself until her next step is so close that it would be on his toes. The leader then uses compression to slow the follower's momentum and push her back to her original position, where she uses an anchor-step to stabilize herself and to prepare for the next basic. Don't worry; you're not supposed to be dancing yet.

> An *anchor-step* is a type of triple-step (counted 1-and-2) that's done in place or slightly backward in the third foot position. West coast swing is the first and only dance in this book that includes an anchor-step.

WCS is considered a dancer's dance due to the complex timing and intricate lead-and-follow details, which we'll cover later in this chapter. The good news is that once you get it, you get it. Let's take a look at how the basic comes together.

West coast swing, in layman's terms, is said out loud like this:

Walk, walk, tap-step, anchor-step,

Walk, walk, tap-step, anchor-step

If you're more mathematically inclined and like to use numbers for your steps, it's counted like this:

One, two, three, four, five-and-six,

One, two, three, four, five-and-six

To gain an appreciation of the right look of a WCS basic, you should picture yourself dancing on a tightrope with the leader staying in place and the follower coming in and then away again in a very repetitive motion. The leader will be in control, but the follower will be the one who gets showcased because all eyes will be on her.

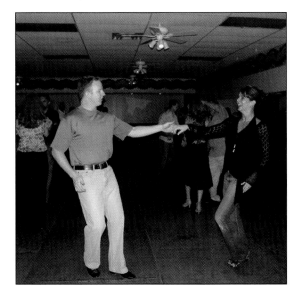

To try the WCS basics in place (you can stand next to one another for this one), assume foot position 1 and be in your respective ready positions. Next, you'll want to simply step down on count 1 (changing weight), then step down on count 2 (again changing weight), then do a tap (just the toe part of your foot, but you won't change weight) on count 3, step down on count 4, then do a triple-step in place on counts 5 and 6. Try them with the counts now, and it'll sound like this: 1, 2, 3, 4, 5-and-6.

Layered Approach to the Basic

Rather than trying to learn everything together at once, it's best to learn WCS in layers. Work on one element, then work your way to the next, and so on. There are several pieces that make up the whole. Followers, these next few paragraphs are mostly for you, but make sure the leaders read along and do the pieces they need to. Each time the follower adds another element, the leader should do the basics in place while the follower is moving beside him. Each of you should go ahead and do your basics one time in place using the timing: 1, 2, 3, 4, 5-and-6, then begin.

Walks

Followers, you get to start out by traveling toward your partner. On the first two counts, take two small steps forward (this will be toward your partner when he's in front of you). Leaders, you'll do your first two counts in place. Do counts 3 through 6 in place and add just this piece. You can both now practice by saying the following: Walk, walk, tap-step in place, and then anchor-step. Followers, you should now find that your starting point is a little farther forward each time you do this.

Taps

To even this out a little bit, followers, you'll now add in a step going backward. On the tap-step, you'll tap slightly forward (just ahead of your left foot or even with it) with your right foot, then step back with your right foot (traveling backward and behind your left foot). Leaders, do your tap-step in place without going anywhere. Counts 5 through 6 remain the same when you go to practice this one. You now have the walk, walk (followers are going forward), tap-step (followers are now heading backward), and then the anchor-step (no movement yet). Followers, you should still end up a little farther forward than where you started at the end of each basic.

Triples

Now, let's finish this by adding in the anchor-step, where counts 5-and-6 are now done slightly backward by the followers in third foot position. Followers, you'll be moving backward because of your momentum. Don't be alarmed by this. Leaders, for now, just go ahead and do a normal triple-step in place. Adding this piece in from the beginning, we now have a complete, mobile basic that has the follower going forward and then backward to her original starting point. At the end of each basic, the follower should be back on her left foot (in third foot position) and ready to step with her right foot. Leaders should be on their right foot and ready to step with their left.

Leaders, while the follower is going back and forth, you should be dancing, for the most part, in place and without a whole lot of motion either way. It might sound a bit strange, but you'll get used to it once you get going on the next part and understand more of the compression and what your roles are for this dance.

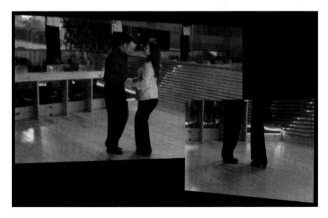

Mirroring

When you're comfortable with the basics in place, go ahead and move into the next part, which will allow you to do the basics of WCS without having to worry about anything but the footwork. In going through your steps this time, stand directly in front of each other. Try facing each other, as shown in the figure below, but be about five feet away from your partner in a mirrored position. It often helps if you're able to see the opposite steps, if for no other reason than to validate your own.

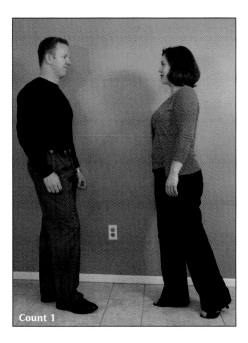

Count 1

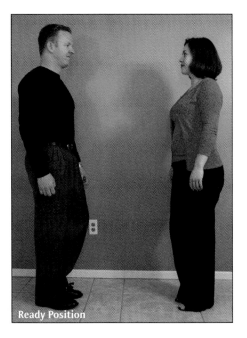

Ready Position

1. (Step 1 - Count 1) From a ready position, leaders will step in place or slightly backward (only a couple of inches at most) with their left foot (second foot position) and followers will step forward with their right foot (fourth foot position) toward the leader, with each partner changing weight to the foot that was moving by the end of step or count 1.

2. (Step 2 - Count 2) Leaders, step in place or slightly backward (again, only a couple of inches at most) with your right foot (second foot position). Followers, step forward with your left foot (fourth foot position) directly toward the leader again. Followers, as you take this second step, turn your left foot slightly to the right as you step so you're at a slight angle, but still coming toward him. This slight angle change will also mean that your left shoulder is now pointed toward the leader and your right shoulder is away from him. Most of the space between the leader and follower disappears once the follower takes her second step. Rather than the five feet of space that you originally had, you should now have about 12 to 18 inches separating the two of you.

3. (Step 3 - Count 3) Leaders, tap your left foot (toes) beside the instep of your right foot, and don't change weight. Followers, tap your

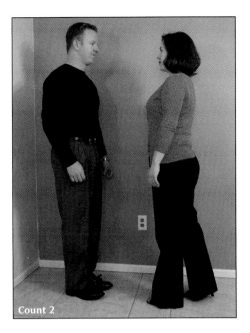

Count 2

4. (Step 4 - Count 4) Leaders, you'll now step in place with your left foot (second foot position) just as you did on the first count (Step 1), except this time, you'll want to step slightly forward because you'll need it to help send the follower the other direction. (You'll learn more about that later in this chapter.) Followers, you'll now step back with your right foot because you're now going to be traveling away from the leader. This step, although you're still slightly angled to your right when you start it, will be in fourth foot position; you'll be squared up with the leader once you take your step.

right foot (toes) beside the instep of your left foot, and don't change weight. The term "beside," as it's used here, means as close to the instep as you can get without stepping on it.

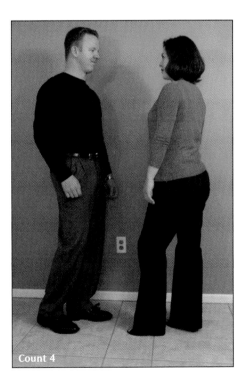

Count 4

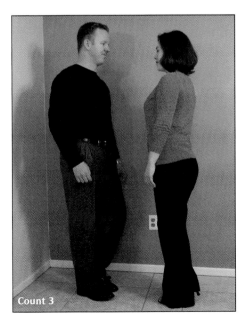

Count 3

Counts 3 and 4 should also be learned using a triple-step. The tap-step is most common for what's called a "sugar push," but the triple-step is regularly substituted here and will be used later in this chapter. Leaders, go ahead and do a triple-step in place or do the 3 and the "and" in third foot position and come back to center for the 4. Followers, you'll step forward with your right on count 3, bring your left foot together on the count "and," and then step back with your right foot on count 4.

5. (Step 5 - Counts 5-and-6) This is that anchor-step we've been telling you about. Leaders, we had you doing a triple-step in place the first time, and now you'll add onto it. You'll do a modified anchor-step in place where your right foot steps back into the fifth foot position on count 5. You do the "and" step in place with your left foot (still in fifth foot position), and then you step out to the right with your right foot into a second foot position. You can say your steps like this: Rock-in place-side, or an-chor-step, or back-and-side, or any combination of three words that fit to help you with these three steps.

Followers, your anchor-step will be just like the one you learned earlier. You'll be traveling backward starting with your left foot in the third foot position. You'll take your left foot back on count 5 into an extended third foot position, then bring your right foot straight back into a third foot position, then end with your left foot going back into an extended third foot position again. Ladies, it's best to say your steps with just the anchor-step naming convention as you practice.

If you executed the steps correctly, you're slightly turned to the left of your partner at the end of the basic, and if you were looking straight ahead, you'd have to turn your head to the right to align with your partner. Did you get it?

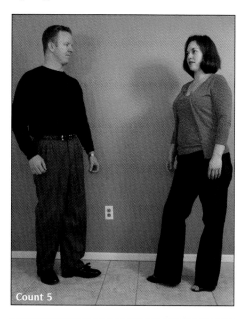

Count 5

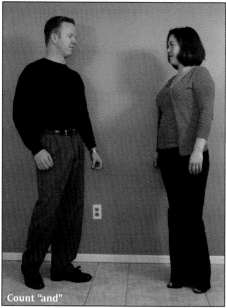

Count "and"

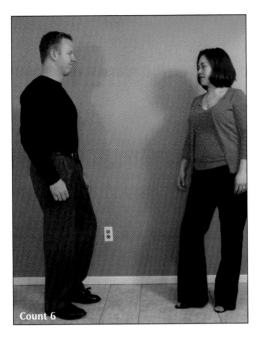

Count 6

It's especially important that at the end of each basic, the followers are on their left foot and they have not started coming forward toward the guys yet. Ladies, you have to wait until count 1 to start coming forward, and that will only be after the guy leads it (once we get to that part). Just make sure you're still traveling away from the guy up through count 6.

When you're both able to do a complete basic on your own, then another, then another, go ahead and practice what you just learned with music. It'll be the last thing you try before you learn to dance it together. Leaders, count out loud to give the follower a chance to match you step for step when you start. The leader should say "Ready, go" or "Ready, and" or even just "5-6-7-8" prior to starting. This should make it easier for both partners.

As always, if either partner gets on the "wrong foot" during the exercise, just stop, laugh, and start up again after the leader counts it off…"Ready, and," and you're back dancing again.

Practice until you're both comfortable with the steps and you know the answers to each of the following questions:

▶ At the end of each basic, should you be in your ready position, second foot position, extended third foot position, or fifth foot position?

▶ Are there any steps that you'll take in a six-count basic that do not include a change of weight?

▶ Who does the majority of traveling during the West coast swing?

▶ Should the ladies be coming forward or going backward on count 6?

▶ Is West coast swing a slotted dance, a circular dance, a stationary dance, or a progressive dance?

▶ How many of the five foot positions are used in the basic?

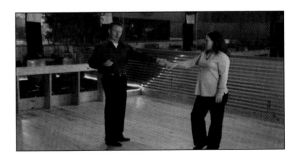

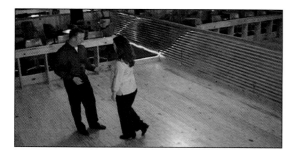

The Six-Count Basic as a Couple

It's more important in WCS than in any other dance that you know your steps individually before trying them with your partner. The leading and following portion of WCS has much detail to it, and you sure don't want to be working on your footwork at the same time. All right, if you're ready, it's now time to get together with your partner and see what happens.

Your toolkit for the WCS basics includes:

- ▶ **Foot position 1 (ready position—to start only, and during tap of the tap-step on count 3)**
- ▶ **Foot position 2 (for leaders on counts 1, 2, 4, and 6 of the basic)**
- ▶ **Foot position 3 (for followers on counts 5-and-6 of the basic; Note: Counts 5, 6 are in extended third)**
- ▶ **Foot position 4 (for followers on counts 1, 2, 4 of the basic)**
- ▶ **Foot position 5 (for leaders on counts 5-and of the basic)**
- ▶ **Connection point 1**
- ▶ **Six-count basic (essential for the WCS to work)**

The Leader's Connector

Go ahead and get into position to start your WCS. The first thing you'll want to do is square up with your partner about four to five feet apart and extend your hand out for connection point 1. Leaders, you'll have your left arm and hand extended at about waist level (your arm is still slightly bent), with your thumb pointing toward 11 o'clock (assuming 12 o'clock is straight up and down) and your fingers creating hook-like fingers (curled fingers) that appear to be pointing back toward yourself. Then, you'll want to take your middle two fingers (your middle and ring fingers) of the four that are hooked and bring them in just a little bit closer to you. (This should now almost look like a sideways "I love you" hand sign from American Sign Language.) Compare your hand with the picture below.

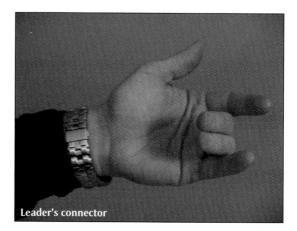

Leader's connector

The Follower's Connector

Ladies, it's your turn. You now get to extend your right arm (slightly bent) and your hand with the intent of connecting on the two fingers that the leader has made the biggest hook with (the middle two of the four). You'll now make that same "I love you" hand sign, but do so with your palm facing the ground. This now separates your middle two fingers (your middle and ring fingers) from the others as well. Are you with me? The thumbs from both the leader and the follower should stay relaxed and uninvolved (no squeezing) as you bring the hands together.

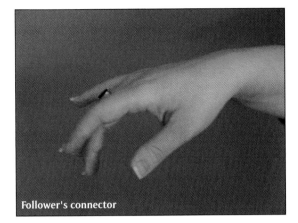

Follower's connector

Connecting the Connectors

Okay, now, ladies, place those two fingers on the inside of the leader's two fingers and wiggle them around a little bit. Both of you should be able to move your fingers around because there should be some play back and forth. Just make sure the fingers are not tense. Now, add a little resistance to the fingers and see whether you can get the leader to pull you closer to him by having him pull his hand and fingers in. If it works, we're ready to go. If not, continue working on it for a few minutes.

The fingers that are not connected (the index finger and pinkie) should not be sticking out like little antennae. Although they're not connected, they need to be relaxed and down near the other fingers, not straight up in the air.

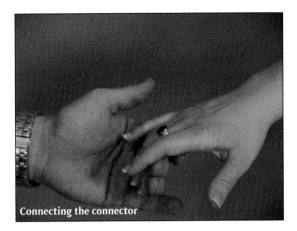

Connecting the connector

Leaders, we're going to work with just this one connection point for a moment and add on so you'll understand its use. Use only your left hand (the follower's right hand) for the next couple of minutes, and we'll let you know when to use your right hand. We'll walk through the basics at the same time so you see where this fits.

Leaders, shift your center point backward while bringing your left hand in toward you on the first count (which also brings the follower toward you) and maintain the same height as it gets closer. Slow your hand down on count 2 as your left elbow gets to your side (don't let it go past your back), and then stop it all together. You should still have the follower's two fingers connected to your two fingers. Yes? No? Well, you should.

Compression

Now start over and do the same exercise, except this time, once you have the follower's momentum coming toward you, let go of the finger-to-finger connection on count 2 and open up your fingers so that your palm is now facing the follower and your fingers are pointing off to the left of her. Followers, your momentum should carry the back of your fingers on your right hand directly into the palm of his left hand by count 3. Ladies, you'll want to press the top side of your fingers into the leader's palm. Your palm should be parallel to the floor with your fingers slightly bent, but pointed straight down so the tops of your fingers between the first and second knuckles are pressing into his palm, not your knuckles alone. This is called *compression*.

> ***Compression*** **describes the process when two bodies or objects are being pressed together using movement, not muscle. In the case of WCS, the leader and the follower are being pressed together at their connection points.**

Leaders, you'll need to slow down the follower's momentum by letting her weight compress into your hand through the count 3-and. To do this, you'll want to extend your left hand toward her slightly, let the backs of her fingers join with your palm, and then bring your hand back toward your body as you slow her down (again, don't let your elbow go past your back). Voila! You have compression! Once you've slowed her forward progress, you'll redirect her weight and send her backward on count 4. When you do this, her hand will separate from your palm for a brief second, and then you'll reconnect the fingers again just before count 5 and make the whole thing seem like it was meant to be. This is tricky!

Leverage

Once the fingers are reconnected on count 5, each partner will slightly extend his or her arms (don't straighten them, though) and do the respective anchor-steps while using leverage.

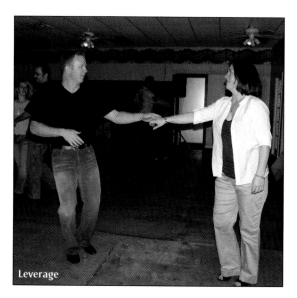
Leverage

> ***Leverage*** **describes the process when two bodies or objects are pulling away from each other using movement, not muscle. In the case of WCS, the leader and the follower are slightly pulling away, almost like the stretching of a rubber band, during the anchor-steps.**

Two-Hand Compression

Go ahead and try to work your way through a couple of basics with just the one hand. Then, leaders, when you're ready, add your right hand into the mix (followers, add your left hand), though it will only get involved for the compression and send off, and then it will disappear again. Leaders, your right hand should be even and at the same height as your left hand. The palm of your right hand should be facing your partner, and your fingers should be aimed toward your partner's feet (at a slight diagonal rather than straight down). Followers, your left hand will compress straight into the leader's right hand, and your fingers should be facing down, just like your right hand is. Compressing into both hands should give the follower a much better sense of balance as she compresses in and then gets sent back, only to reconnect with her right hand on counts 5-and-6.

After you understand each of the pieces, you can logically break the basic West coast swing steps down into three main parts:

1. Walk
2. Compress
3. Anchor

Leaders, you can say these three pieces out loud as you bring the follower back and forth. To practice the six-count basic, one could easily use the phrase "walk - compress - anchor," and then "walk - compress - anchor," and so on.

Practice, Practice, Practice

Okay, leaders, go ahead and give your starting count of "Ready, and," and step slightly back with your left and then with your right, compress during the tap-step, send the follower away, and do the anchor-step. Now that you got through one basic, repeat it over and over.

It's more than likely going to take some practice to make it look and feel natural! Don't sweat it—this is not an easy dance to master, and almost everyone goes through the same learning curve. Sure, the basics seem easy enough on their own, but if you really want to be a great lead-and-follow WCS dancer, understanding the physics behind each and every step and count is a must.

Go ahead and dance through the WCS basics a few times. It should be working by now. Is it? If so, you did or felt each of the following (you should aim for at least five of the six):

▶ **You successfully completed all six counts.**

▶ **You both felt completely overwhelmed with all the details, but you understand the logic.**

▶ **You managed to stay directly in front of one another.**

▶ **You felt a bit uncoordinated, yet more intelligent for understanding.**

▶ **You both had a smile on your face or caused one with your perplexed look.**

▶ **You weren't satisfied with the basic, but you were optimistic because you're getting better.**

Value of the Basic

What you just learned in this chapter about the basic will apply to every move in WCS that you'll learn from here on out. Guys, the more you understand how to manipulate the woman's momentum, movement, and positioning through your lead, the better off you'll be. Ladies, the more you know about what feels right and why, the better you'll be in following because you'll know how to compensate when needed and you'll know when to just sit back and enjoy the dance naturally.

As more moves and patterns are added into your repertoire, you'll find that they all have the same basic components, such as the walking-steps, tap-steps, triple-steps, and anchor-steps. The walking-steps and anchor-steps can be found in almost every pattern, but the tap-step won't. As mentioned earlier in the chapter, the tap-steps can be interchanged with triple-steps during the basic, and triple-steps are almost always used in place of the tap-steps when patterns require the leader and follower to change positions on the slot. You'll get a chance to try a few of these out in the drills that are coming up next.

Fun Drills to Put It All Together

W E'VE PUT TOGETHER a number of fun drills and exercises for you to go through to work on your West coast swing. Instead of just picturing yourself doing the WCS, you've now put it all together and are dancing it for yourself. Go through each of the drills as they focus on different moves, leads, and thinking patterns. Soon, you'll feel confident enough to try your WCS anywhere.

Drill 1: Shadow Dancing

Set up in your ready position in your dance frame and do the basics on your own. Have your partner do his or hers as well, just not with you. Turn some music on and dance through the basics. See who can last the longest without messing up, stopping, or getting off beat. Basically, both of you will be WCS dancing individually, running through the leads and/or follows and footwork for all of the steps to music to help get them into your long-term memory.

© istockphoto.com/
Paul Piebinga

Drill 2: The Triple-Tap Swap

Remember the part about triple-steps and tap-steps, and how they're interchangeable on counts 3 and 4? Here's where you get to practice.

Dance the basics five times in a row using the tap-steps, and then stop. Then dance basics five times in a row using the triple-steps and stop again. When you start dancing the third set of five basics, do either the tap-steps or triple-steps in any order you choose, but don't tell your partner which one you're going to do. The object here is to know that either one can and will be used in the basic. Ladies, doing the triple-step more often than not will increase your odds of being ready for any additional moves that are thrown at you.

> **Leaders, for fun, and after you've completed this exercise, see whether you can figure out a way to actually lead the follower into doing one or the other: tap-steps or triple-steps. It's possible, but takes a lot of work—test it and see!**

Drill 3: Hands Solo

This is a fun exercise that uses only one hand at a time, yet it still touches on every bit of the fundamentals. Earlier in the chapter the leader used just his left hand and the follower used just her right hand. For this one, each partner will use both of their hands, just not at the same time. It will test the coordination and timing of each partner.

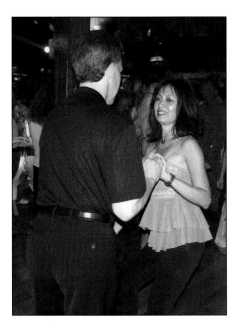

Leaders, start out by using your left hand the way you normally would for counts 1 and 2. Then, on count 3 (it's easiest if you both use triple-steps, but the tap-step can also work), let go of your left hand completely and use only your right hand for the compression through count 4. Then, use just your left hand to reconnect for the anchor-step on counts 5-and-6. The goal is to not disrupt the follower's momentum or pace and to keep her completely within your control, even though you're changing your hands out at a rapid pace. Leaders, once you master this one, you can easily add it into your normal dance routine because it's a fun way to do the basics with others.

Drill 4: Four Square

Not what you think here, but along the same lines. This drill reinforces the leader's ability to stay within his boundaries. To keep the leader constrained to movement, practice on a floor that has approximately 12-inch square tiles (15-inch ones will work too). Pick any four of the tiles that make up one larger square and have the leader stand in the

crossing of the middle of them. Dance through the basics for a song or two and see whether the leader can stay within that box. Most leaders have a tendency to go either forward or backward an inch or two every basic, so this helps provide a reference for the movement. The goal for the leaders is to end up in the same cross-point in which they started the dance.

> If you don't have a tile floor or something equivalent, you can mark off an area using six pieces of masking tape— one for each of the four sides of the larger square and then a cross-like figure in the middle to separate them.

Drill 5: Dancing with the Fridge

This is a great exercise for the followers. Ladies, this is a chance for you to practice your moving basic without your dance partner—take the time to get extra smooth for the dance floor. What you need is a fridge with handles you can loop a towel through, a small bath towel, and yourself. Loop the towel through the handle, hold on with your right hand, and practice your basics. Lean into the fridge

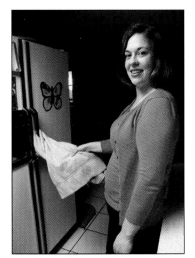

on count 3, and if you open the fridge door on count 4, 5, "and," or 6, you've taken too big of steps back or you've moved too quickly. Practice holding the towel at different lengths to increase the control of your step size.

Hot Tips for the West Coast Swing

FOLLOWING ARE a number of excellent tips, pointers, and reminders for West coast swing dancers now that you're off and looking good on the dance floor. Keep these in mind as you practice your steps.

- ▶ The lead should be on the first count of the basic only; then let momentum, connection, compression, and leverage take over. If the lead is on every count or step, it's no different than dragging, pushing, or pulling someone through an entire dance.

- ▶ Leaders, keep your hands level. The more you move your hands up and down, the harder it is for the follower to key in on your lead.

- ▶ Size matters when it comes to steps, followers. If you take very small steps in this dance, you'll find that it's nothing more than standing in place and moving your feet. If you take too large of steps, you will break the connection with your partner and ruin the momentum. Your movement should be like an accordion that compresses into your partner and then opens back up again.

- ▶ Neither partner should ever fully straighten his or her arms during extension. By the same token, elbows should not pass either person's torso during compression. Elasticity is imperative.

- ▶ WCS is a smooth dance, so keep the lilt, bopping, and bouncing out of the dance and in the regular swing where it belongs.

- ▶ An anchor-step is not intended to pull your partner over; it's there to let you settle into and finish a move or pattern.

- ▶ Squeezing with your thumb (either of you) is unacceptable, unless it's used to assist with a lead. Thumb-squeezing is usually a result of incorrect finger connection, and there's no freedom of motion due to the clamping feeling. Also, it's easy to bruise the back of a hand by squeezing the thumb.

- ▶ Tap-steps and triple-steps for counts 3 and 4 are usually interchangeable because they both result in stepping with the same foot at the end.

- ▶ Don't keep your body perfectly square with the slot at all times. Try to use the different foot positions to open your hips and shoulders. Doing this will also make your dance look much larger than it is. A perfectly squared dancer is typically not much fun to watch.

- ▶ Compression and leverage are results of motion, not of strength. WCS is not the place to demonstrate how strong a lead you have or how quickly you can push/pull someone around.

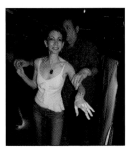

Review and Next Steps for Your West Coast Swing

WOOHOO! That's it! You now have the tools to master the basics of West coast swing. Now, to ensure you're comfortable with the WCS, we're going to run back through the major points of what you've learned and do a final recap.

Review

1. Ladies are always right! Ladies, put your weight on your left foot so you can be ready to start with your right. (In other words, get into your ready position.)

2. Guys always get what's left. Guys, put your weight on your right foot so you can be ready to start with your left. (In other words, get into your ready position.)

3. Connection point 1 (one- or two-hand hold) is used in the basics of WCS.

4. The WCS basic consists of a total of six counts and can be done with a tap-step on counts 3, 4 or a triple-step on 3-and-4.

5. The first walking-step for the leader is the one that travels slightly backward. This helps move his center back, which in turn helps get the follower moving forward.

6. Anchor-steps for the ladies are done with an extended third foot position, then a third, then an extended third again, leaving her left foot (where her weight is) slightly angled at the end of the basic to add some shape and styling to the dance.

7. The two fingers that house the majority of the leading and following in WCS are the middle finger and the ring finger—thumbs should not be used.

8. Compression and leverage are gradual results of motion.

Next Steps

Upon mastering the elasticity of such a cool dance, you're bound to want more. The neat part about WCS is that the basics are but one element of the many different pieces that make up the whole. WCS is unique in that the social lead-and-follow elements of the dance can easily incorporate a six-count pattern, an eight-count pattern, a 10- or 12-count pattern, and then another six-count pattern. Each one is different and can have its own timing and footwork, yet almost all of them start with the walking-steps in some fashion and end with the anchor-step.

To add onto your WCS, you'll want to visit a local class or instructor in your area. WCS dancers and social clubs have one of the largest followings of any of the dance types. Take a look online for the group nearest you that matches your interests. The best part about WCS is that you can dance it for much longer periods than other types of swing due to its slower rhythm. You don't typically feel like you're going to die after a couple of West coast swings. Dress casually and head on out to the dance floor. A good time awaits you!

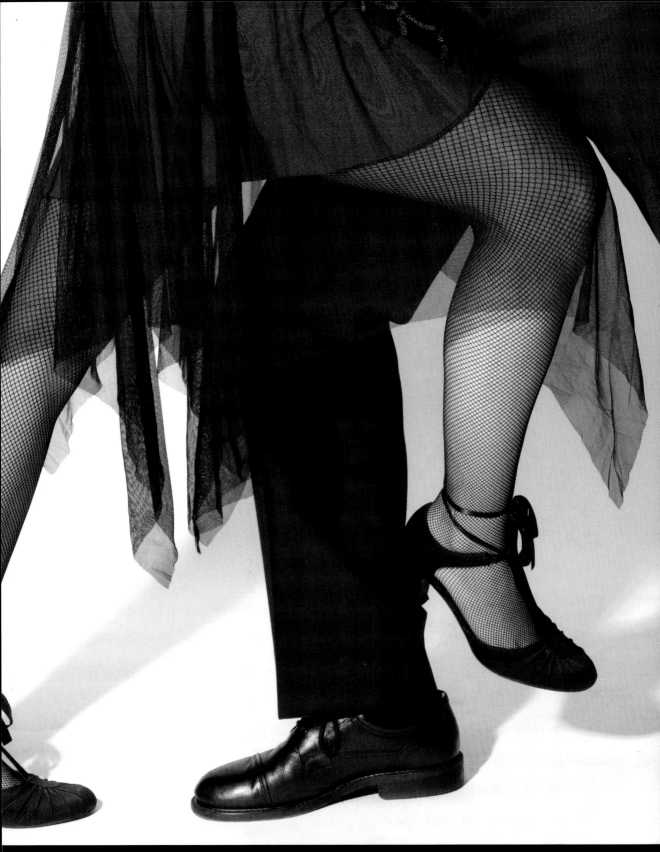

11

Picture Yourself

Dancing

the Tango

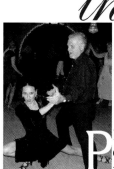

PICTURE YOURSELF striding down the line of dance, cheek to cheek with your partner. Suddenly, as the music cues it, you both stop as if on a dime and rapidly break your progression with a turn. A story of a torrid affair full of passion and desire is told on the dance floor. As you boldly step through the T-A-N-G-O rhythm, you and your partner move your way back through time to the dance's roots in the nightlife of Buenos Aires, Argentina. As a leader you are dancing the story of a man who is tied to his partner by his passion and desire, but a connection at the heart is not necessarily part of the equation. As a follower, you are dancing a dance of fire, with a strong counter for every step offered by the lead. As your skill level increases, you will experience moves of increasing dependence on the leader, such as leans and dramatic dips, but you will also learn patterns of movement that curtly answer a guide from your leader, seemingly taking the wind from his sails. As you master the tango, you and your partner will learn that this dance is a dance of street smarts, even in its most domesticated American style, and even though you can take the tango out of the city, you can never completely remove the city from the tango.

The Six Ws of Tango

T HE TANGO as a dance typifies the romance, passion, and mystery that draw people the world over to couples dancing as a pastime and sport.

Who Created and Popularized the Tango?

The tango was created by African and European immigrants in the slums and working-class neighborhoods of Buenos Aires, Argentina. The dance was born when a new musical style evolved from Argentine, African, French, Indian, and Latin rhythms. From here, the tango was exported to the stages and salons of Europe and the United States. The tango has been popularized and re-popularized over the decades by various movies, both American

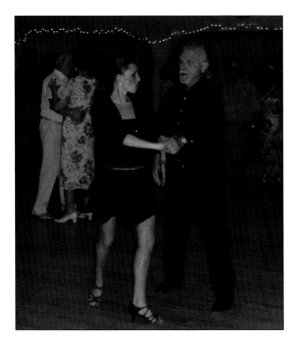

and European, featuring the dance in its original Argentine version or its tamed American or international style.

What Is the Tango?

There are several different types of tango, including Argentine, American, international, Finnish, Chinese, and ballroom styles. The original Argentine tango is a combination of the Argentine polka and an Afro-Argentine dance called the *Candombe*. The tango borrowed the close upper-body hold, hand placement on the waist, and the heel and toe work from the polka and merged it with the knee dips, hip twists, and long, low walking-steps of the Candombe. The early version was known as the *Canyengue*, which then eventually grew into the tango. Although the original music for the tango was written in 2/4 time, the tango music of today is 4/4 time.

The American tango, which is taught in this text, is a strong, rhythmic, progressive dance.

A *progressive dance* describes any dance in which the partners dance around the perimeter of the dance floor in a counterclockwise direction. All of the turns, spins, and other moves are done while the partners are progressing around the floor.

The American social tango focuses on posture, frame, and staccato movement with an emphasis on the partners' respective leading and following skills.

Where Did the Tango Originate and Where Is It Typically Done?

As previously mentioned, tango was born in the heart of Buenos Aires, Argentina. From there, various styles and forms of it spread around the world. Some of these versions were in a sense "exported" by Argentina through stage shows and movies, but the majority of the rest were adapted following export. The American social tango was born when American dance instructors adapted the highly intricate Argentine tango for the less adept American dancing public. The English took the Argentine tango and created the international style, which they adapted for showcase performance and competition. The Argentines maintained the integrity of the Argentine tango over the years by keeping the original tango upper-body positioning and smooth, cat-like steps.

Tango has found a home in ballrooms around the world. Although the tango is not often seen on the American social dance floor outside of the ballroom, this is most often a function of music selection rather than distaste. Tango music has a highly distinctive rhythmic pattern and a heavy beat that is not frequently heard in today's popular music.

When Did the Tango Become Popular and When Is the Right Time to Tango?

The tango was born in the late nineteenth century on the streets of Buenos Aires. The name *tango* was applied to the dance around 1890. The dance was exported to Europe in the early years of the twentieth century through the dancers and orchestras from Buenos Aires. There have been a series of

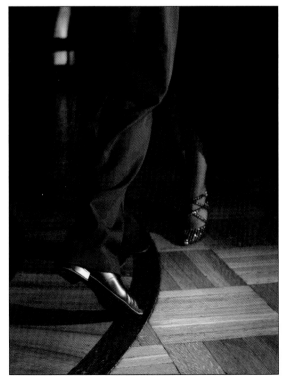

© istockphoto.com/Michal Kozlowski

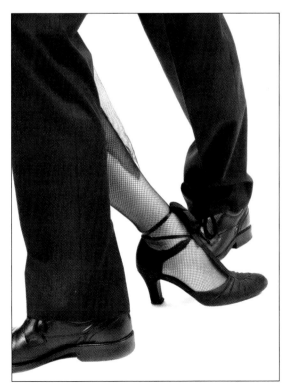

© istockphoto.com/Paul Piebinga

tango crazes over the years, the first of which was in Paris, and which then spread to London, Berlin, and the other capitals of Europe. The tango did not reach the United States until 1913 in New York City, where it became immensely popular. The fortunes of the tango traced the fortunes of Argentina as a country through the twentieth century, with a dramatic slump during the Great Depression and Hipólito Yrigoyen regime. However, tango's golden age is considered to be under the governance of Juan Peron, when the tango was a matter of national pride and immense popularity. However, the popularity of the tango outside of the ballroom once again declined with economic depression and military dictatorships. The tango did not emerge again as an international movement until the 1980s, when tango hit the stage in Paris and on Broadway. Since then, it has remained in the public eye in film and on stage as a passionate icon of couples dance.

The music dictates the dance when it comes to tango, regardless of style. The American social tango is designed to embellish a very specific genre of music that is not often played outside of ballrooms.

Why Is the Tango Danced?

The tango evolved as a dance that showcased the man's ability to lead his partner around the dance floor and through the dance. The American tango is a demonstration of the establishment of this lead and the struggle between the wills of the leader and the follower. The Argentine-style tango expresses the tit for tat exchange between the leader and follower, who are completely attuned to the other's body and movements.

What Kind of Attire Should Be Worn?

There is no dress code for tango dancing. The best guide is to dress for the type of event you will be attending. However, because this dance is almost exclusively danced in the ballroom, wear business-casual clothing for lessons and take your wardrobe cues from your fellow students and your instructors when it comes to social events.

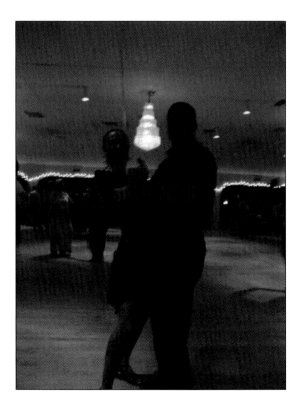

Visualize the Tango

BEFORE EACH LESSON plan, we recommend you take a few minutes or so to watch the accompanying *Couples Ultimate Dance Sampler* DVD. Because tango was added as a bonus chapter, there is not a section on the DVD that covers it in depth. To give yourself a sneak peek at what you'll be learning, you might want to take a few minutes to find a beginner tango clip online— or you can just see whether we can provide you with the visual you'll need just by reading the following sections. We'll do our best to make it as descriptive as possible to give you a good feel for what you're learning and to get you dancing quickly.

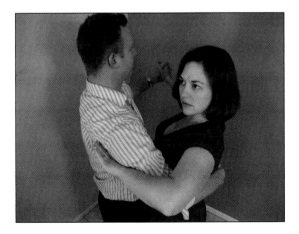

For tango, it will be best for you to skim through the chapter to get the highlights of the material in order to give your mind a chance to get familiar with the dance. Take a look at how the dancers are positioned in the pictures, think about the words that are used, and picture yourself dancing the tango.

As you read through the chapter, you'll still want to take notes on the important parts of the tango so you can engage other parts of the kinesthetic learning prior to getting up and dancing along. Keep track of what the connection points are, what the basic steps are called, how many counts are in a basic, how to align with your partner, and so on. Also, write down any questions that you might have about the tango. There's a good chance you will find the answer later on in this chapter, and if it's something you're already pondering, you'll be sure to remember the answer.

You'll find that by time you get ready to stand up and try the tango, the dancing won't be nearly as overwhelming. Writing down the key concepts will allow you to get a jumpstart on the rest of this chapter. You'll find that after you get up and try it, you'll probably have more questions. As this chapter goes on, the steps will be broken out with pictures depicting both the leader's part and the follower's part, pointers will be given on where you should be during different parts of the dance, and frequently asked questions will be addressed that should satisfy most, if not all, of your questions and then some.

Just remember, everyone learns at a different pace. Be cognizant of this as you're learning with your partner. One of you might pick up certain aspects of the tango quicker than the other, and that's okay. Try to be patient and wait for the other person to grasp the material, and then move on.

Now, take a look at the pictures below. All of them are taken of couples dancing the tango. Some are formal, some are very informal, but they're all doing the same steps. See whether you can visualize yourself dancing the tango in all these different settings. Then, picture yourself dancing the tango at upcoming events or at local venues where you and your partner can go. Any idea where you will go out dancing after you learn the tango?

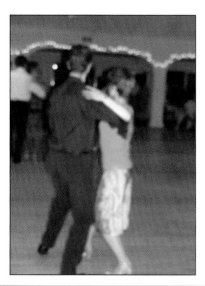

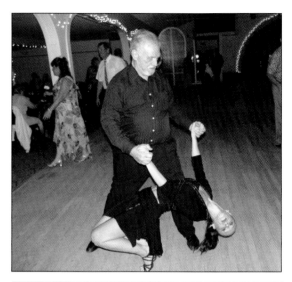

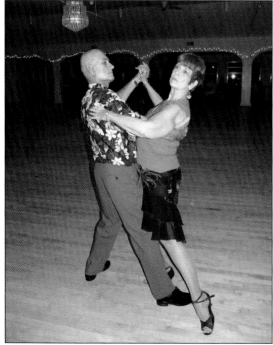

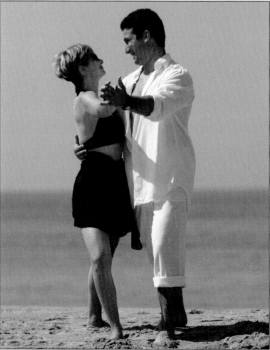

© **istockphoto.com/Galina Barskaya**

Tango Basics

TANGO IS ONE OF THE few dances that really fits the music. The major beats in tango music allow the dancer to easily follow along and invoke a wide array of emotions, including passion, excitement, tenderness, sadness, love, romance, and anger. Tango can best be described as a smooth, progressive, and theatrical dance that has both partners doing cat-like or stalking walks with knees that are continuously flexed.

The smooth part of tango means that there should not be any rise and fall because the dancers' bodies should remain at a constant level throughout the dance. Progressive means the dancers will be moving around the dance floor rather than staying in one central place, such as in swing. The theatrical part of tango is based on the idea that tango has long been recognized as a dance with strong, showy leads, animated facial expressions, and quick and deliberate head movements.

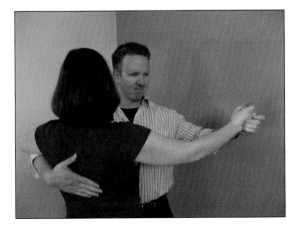

Tango styles vary and include Argentine, Gaucho, French, international, and many others. The style you're learning here is the American version, which includes the best parts of each. The tango basic is eight counts full of sharp, deliberate steps in which the body moves directly over the feet and at the same time. When your feet stop moving, so should your body. The basics include walking-steps, side-steps, and a close (tap-step with hold) to both slow and quick timings.

> Walking-steps are done to both slow and quick rhythms in the basic, side-steps are quick, and the close is done slow with the tap on one count and a hold (no movement) on the second.

As previously mentioned, the tango is danced to 4/4 timing, which means the number of songs you can practice to is quite extensive, though for very pronounced tango rhythms it's best to do a search for "tango music" online and pick from whatever genre of music fits your style the best. Once you hear a good tango, there'll be no doubt in your mind what one should include, and you'll easily be able to recognize the music and be ready to dance when the opportunity arises. Before we begin the tango, let's recap our two most important rules:

1. Ladies are always right! Ladies, put your weight on your left foot so you can be ready to start with your right. (This is what's called your *ready position.*)

2. Guys always get what's left. Guys, put your weight on your right foot so you can be ready to start with your left. (This is what's called your *ready position.*)

The Eight-Count Basic

The eight-count progressive basic of tango is made up of three walking-steps, a side-step, and a close (similar to a tap-step with a hold). The term "progressive" is used because the dancers dance counterclockwise around the dance floor with gradual turns off to the left during the walking-steps.

To give you a mental image of the dance, tango starts out with the leaders and followers standing in a tightly closed and more compact dance frame (more than any other dance in this book), completely offset so there's no chance of stepping on one another's feet on the first step. The follower's left hand (connection point 4) is modified and is now firmly positioned underneath the leader's right arm with the follower's palm facing inward. The dancers start the dance by taking slow, steady jungle cat–like steps, and then rushing off to the side to gain a new perspective on their prey. And then they stop . . . only to hold for a brief second and then begin again.

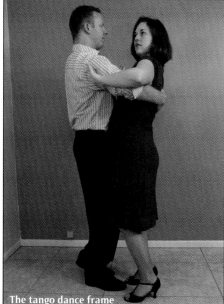
The tango dance frame

Tango is not as much a social dance as it is an exhibition dance, due to its show qualities. However, it's up to you as the dancer to develop the strong sense of connection with the music, your partner, and the audience to pull off this dance. It's important in tango that you feel the music and project your emotions outward.

Tango, in layman's terms, is said out loud like this:

Walk, walk, walk, side, together (or close)

Walk, walk, walk, side, together (or close)

An easy way to remember and practice these steps later is to use the following phrase while dancing the basics: "Walk, walk, tan-go-close," where the "tan-go-close" means step, side, together.

If you're more mathematically inclined and like to use numbers for your steps, it's counted like this:

One......three......five...six...seven......one......three......five...six...seven......

> **Just remember, there's no change of weight on the last step in tango. Whether you say it as "Together" or "Close" or "7" or the letter "O," as you'll learn about in a moment, you need to be sure not to change weight during the basics.**

And now, two classic teaching methods for learning the tango: Replace the counts with slow and quick steps, or replace both the steps and counts with the letters of the word "tango," done to the same timing.

**Slow......slow......quick...quick...slow......slow......
slow......quick...quick...slow......**

or

**T(1)......A(3)......N(5)...G(6)...O(7)......T......A......
N...G...O......**

(The numbers next to the letters represent the
count you'd use for each step.)

To try the tango basics in place (you can stand next
to one another for this one), assume foot position
1, and be in your respective ready positions. Next,
you'll want to simply step down on count 1
(changing weight, then holding for a count), then
step down on count 3 (again changing weight and
holding for a count), then step down and change
weight rapidly on counts 5 and 6, then do a tap on
7 and hold count 8 with no stepping or motion.
Try these steps with each type of the basic counts,
and you'll have the following: "Walk, walk, tan-go-
close," or "1...3...5, 6, 7," or "Slow, slow, quick, quick,
slow," or the letters "T...A...N-G-O."

Mirroring

When you're comfortable stepping in place, go
ahead and move into the next part, which will
allow you to do the basics of tango without having
to worry about anything but the footwork. In
going through your steps this time, stand directly
in front of one another and be about five feet away
in a mirrored position. It often helps if you're able
to see the opposite steps, if for no other reason
than to validate your own.

1. **T** *slow* (Step 1 - Counts 1 and 2) From a ready
   position, leaders will step forward with their
   left foot (fourth foot position), and followers
   will step backward with their right foot
   (fourth foot position) away from the leader,
   with each partner changing weight to the
   foot that was moving on count 1. This is
   nothing more than a walking-step with very
   pronounced steps (no sliding or gliding
   during tango).

2. **A** *slow* (Step 2 - Counts 3 and 4) Leaders will
   step forward again, but this time with their
   right foot (fourth foot position), and followers will step backward with their left foot
   (fourth foot position) away from the leader,
   with each partner changing weight to the
   foot that was moving on count 3. This is the
   same kind of walking-step as in Step 1.

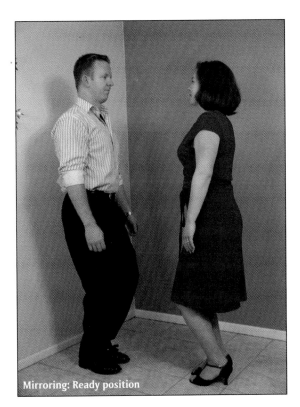

Mirroring: Ready position

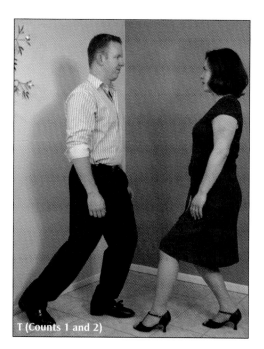

T (Counts 1 and 2)

3. N *quick* (Step 3 - Count 5) Leaders will step front-left this time with their left foot (extended third foot position), and followers will step back-right with their right foot, with each partner changing weight to the foot that was moving on count 5. The importance of this step is that it lets the leaders gradually turn to the left and it positions him for easy transitions into corners. A sharper step left by the leader results in a much more abrupt turn, whereas a step forward (not angled) results in a basic that never turns.

4. G *quick* (Step 4 - Count 6) Leaders will step to the right with their right foot (second foot position), and followers will step left with their left foot (second foot position), with each partner changing weight to the foot that was moving on count 6. This side-step is relative to the positioning of the foot after Step 3 - Count 5 because the foot should be in second foot position on count 6.

5. O *slow* (Step 5 - Counts 7 and 8) Leaders, close your left foot next to your right foot and do a tap on count 7. Followers, close your right next to your left and do a tap with it as well. Make sure you're both in foot position

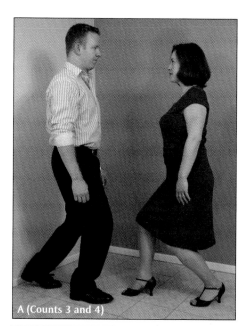

A (Counts 3 and 4)

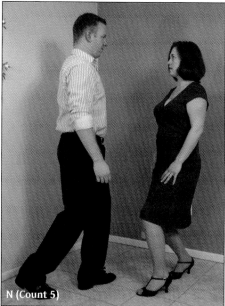

N (Count 5)

one (your ready position) and that neither of you changes weight when you close your feet. Also, there's no movement or change of weight on the count 8 because it's the final count before starting over.

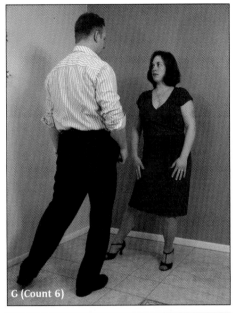

G (Count 6)

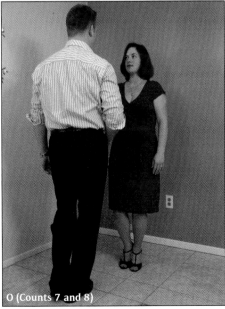

O (Counts 7 and 8)

When you're both able to do a complete tango basic on your own, and then several more without any problems, go ahead and practice what you just learned with music. It'll be the last thing you try before you learn to dance it together. Leaders, count out loud to give the follower a chance to match you step for step when you start. The leader should say "Ready, go" or "Ready, and" just prior to starting to make it easier for both partners.

> As always, if either partner gets on the "wrong foot" during practice, just stop, laugh, and start again after the leader counts it off. . . . "Ready, and," and you're back dancing again.

Practice until you're both comfortable with the steps and you know the answers to each of the following questions:

- ▶ At the end of each basic, should you be in your ready position, the second foot position, extended third foot position, or fifth foot position?

- ▶ Are there any steps that you'll take in an eight-count basic that do not include a change of weight? If so, which ones?

- ▶ Does either partner move more than the other during the tango?

- ▶ Should the ladies be coming forward, going backward, or heading left on count 6?

- ▶ Is tango a stationary dance, a circular dance, a slotted dance, or a progressive dance?

- ▶ How many of the five foot positions are used in the basic?

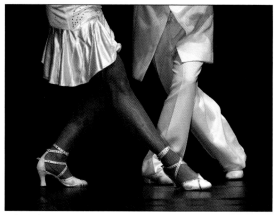

© istockphoto.com/Daniel Ruta

The Eight-Count Basic as a Couple

It's critical that you know your basic in tango before coming together. Being as close as you are to start with, it's very easy to get stepped on or run over if you don't know your steps. The leading and following portion of social tango mostly deals with body positioning and movement, rather than strong arm or finger leads. Now, if you're ready, it's now time to pair up with your partner and give it a shot.

Your toolkit for the tango basics includes:

- ▶ Foot position 1 (ready position to start the dance and during the tap on count 7)

- ▶ Foot position 2 (count 6)

- ▶ Foot position 3 (extended third on count 5 for gradual left turn)

- ▶ Foot position 4 (counts 1 and 3 of the basic; on count 5 if there's no gradual left turn)

- ▶ Connection points 1–4 (modified connection point 4)

- ▶ Eight-count basic (essential for the tango to work)

Reconstructing the Frame

To construct the proper look of the tango, it's important to rebuild what you've already mastered in the other dances. There are a few differences in tango, primarily due to the closeness or distance between you and your partner.

First, you'll need to stand no more than about two feet apart and get into your regular dance frame using all four connection points. Now you'll want to move in as close as you can get without stepping on one another and without your bodies getting too close for comfort. (Make sure you're offset.) If you're in closer than you have been in any of the other dances (except for maybe the slow dance), then you probably noticed that connection point 1 had to extend out to the side in order to maintain the frame.

> Be sure to keep your head up and look slightly to the left. If you look slightly right, you'd be looking at one another, which is contrary to the style guidelines of American tango.

Connection point 2, leaders, now will change, and your right hand will go toward the middle of her back at a downward-sloping angle with a nice straight line. Leaders, your right wrist/forearm will now cross over the follower's shoulder blade (scapula) and your fingers will rest near the follower's spine.

Connection point 4, followers, will have your left hand and forearm around the back of the leader's right arm with your wrist directly underneath his arm and your palm facing inward (toward you at an angle). This connection helps give the look of tango, regardless of whether you're doing the correct footwork.

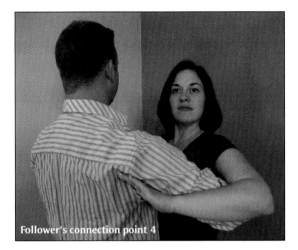

Follower's connection point 4

Practicing the Basics

Now that you've got the right connection points and you know the footwork, it's time to give it a try. You should practice until both of you are comfortable with the steps and no one is getting stepped on. Try to dance in a straight line, and then around corners as needed. The majority of the lead is through the leader's center point, so make sure it's not all being led with the hands. In tango, just like in every other dance, the follower should feel as though her body is completely controlled by the leader, especially because the frame has the dancers much closer. The lead should be so clear that the follower could literally do the steps blindfolded.

> Practicing with the follower blindfolded (or with her eyes closed) is great for testing the leader's command of the dance as well as the follower's reception. The follower being blindfolded should have no impact on the couple's success on the dance floor. She should be able to do every step without using her eyes.

The more time you spend on the basics, the better off you'll be. If there's a part you don't understand or one that just simply isn't working, you might want to contact a local professional to get it worked out. Success is marked when everything is working together and both partners are moving effortlessly around the dance floor with one another. We'll add in a number of fun variations for you to work further with the tango rhythm. See whether you can follow along as we go, because this is where your thinking skills will have to take over. Enjoy!

Fun Drills to Put It All Together

THIS SECTION will be great fun for you as you work your way through the exercises while reinforcing the key elements of the chapter. Instead of just picturing yourself dancing tango, it's time to put it all together and add on to it. Go through each drill as they focus on different moves, leads, and thinking patterns.

Drill 1: T-A-NGO

Set up in your ready position with your hands extended as though your partner is connected, but do the basics on your own. Have your partner do his or hers as well, just not with you; your partner will be a couple of feet away. Speak the letters T-A-NGO out loud together in a rhythm that sounds like the popular children's song B-I-NGO (you know, ". . . and Bingo was his name-o!") and dance through the basics repetitively. Each walking-step should be both bold and firm. See who can last the longest without messing up, stopping, or getting off beat.

Drill 2: It Takes Two to Tango

Set up in your ready position, but this time with your partner, and practice the basics of tango to several different speeds. No music is necessary, but it can certainly help. Practice slowly, at normal speed (normal is what you feel most comfortable with), and then as fast as you can handle. Test your limits and try to hold each slow to the very last second before moving.

Drill 3: Flying off the Handle

A great way to learn or practice the turning basics and basic tango rhythm (either for going around corners or just to do a complete basic in a circular fashion) is to use a broomstick. (And it's fun, too!) This is one you can do on your own or with your partner. Place the broomstick out to where connection point 1 would be and let it stand vertically so the broom handle is at the top. Use only 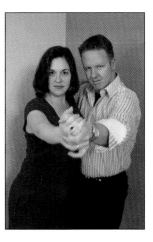 connection point 1, but do so by placing your hand around the handle. Now, leaders, you'll be going forward and your steps will be rounded to the left. Followers, you'll be traveling backward and to your right. After you're finished practicing this one with the broomstick, try it with your partner and see whether you can do the same type of turns.

Drill 4: Rockin' Out

Another fun and easy way to increase your mobility on the tango floor is to add rock-steps into your basic. Set up in your ready position with your partner and begin to do the basics. Rather than doing two walking-steps forward on the first two steps (counts 1–4), you'll do a rock-step. Then, leaders, you'll step and turn approximately a quarter turn to your left (and take the follower with you) on the next count (5), before stepping to the side for a normal close. Essentially, this one is rock-step, turn, side, close. Replacing the walking-steps on this one will enable the leaders to add more into their basic and be able to turn quickly if there's a reason not to go straight down the line of dance.

Hot Tips for the Tango

TANGO IS and always will be in a class by itself among the social dances. Very few dances can even come close to evoking the same type of emotional whirlwind as the tango. Following are a number of tips, pointers, and reminders for how to make tango into one of your favorite dances, as well as a favorite for your audience. Keep each tip in mind as you practice your dance and prepare for your exhibition.

▶ **Each walking-step should be bold, firm, and in control.**

▶ **The tango basics are the most important. Do them well, and you'll be able to do almost anything out on the social dance floor. Practice the tango basics until they become second nature.**

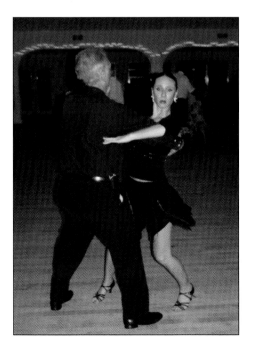

▶ **It's very important to hold each slow to the very last second before moving.**

▶ **Avoid putting any rise and fall or any other body motion or flight into your tango.**

▶ **Flexed knees are a must. For the correct look and feel of the tango, it's imperative that you feel as though you're down into your knees, yet standing tall and completely balanced (both of you).**

▶ **Stay close to your partner. The tango closed dance position is closer than the closed position in many other dances and requires a modified dance position.**

▶ **Do not blend steps! Whether quicks or slows, your steps should be clearly defined, should not be blended into one another, and must contain a transfer of weight when appropriate as well as a clearly defined hold on the final step.**

▶ **Dance tango the way it's described— smooth, progressive, and theatrical.**

▶ **Add emotion into your dance. Tango can easily incorporate emotions such as passion, excitement, tenderness, sadness, love, romance, and anger. Try practicing each one while you're dancing.**

▶ **Keep your head up, your upper body fairly firm, and your connections intact. This will help your control over each step as you dance the tango.**

▶ **When your feet stop moving, so should your body!**

Review and Next Steps for Your Tango

YOU'RE NOW ON the verge of tango completeness. To wrap up the tango, we'll do a final review to make sure you're comfortable with the major concepts and points. Again, go through each one and come back to this list as necessary for a quick review. Start at the beginning and work your way through each point.

Review

1. Ladies are always right! Ladies, put your weight on your left foot so you can be ready to start with your right. (In other words, get into your ready position.)

2. Guys always get what's left. Guys, put your weight on your right foot so you can be ready to start with your left. (In other words, get into your ready position.)

3. All four connection points are used in the basics of the tango. Just remember, connection points 2 and 4 are modified to fit the closeness of the dance.

4. There are at least four fun ways to count the basics: "Walk, walk, tan-go-close," "1...3...5, 6, 7," "Slow, slow, quick, quick, slow," and the letters "T, A, N-G-O."

5. Rock-steps can replace the walking-steps in a basic to allow for a stationary movement or to start a turn in place.

6. Turning corners should be gradual and spaced out, almost as if you are making a very large circle. Small, tight circles can also be executed on a much more infrequent basis by using tight, rounded steps, as you learned with the broom handle.

7. Flexed knees; smooth, deliberate steps; good posture; and emotion-filled expressions are all great characteristics of the tango and should be incorporated into every basic.

Next Steps

Now that you've completed the tango, did you find that it can be fun to learn because the musical beats are easy to recognize and follow? Are you ready to continue learning the tango? Tango has become more and more popular among social dance clubs and has always been a staple in the ballroom studios. To find more information about the tango, there are many directions you can go. Whether it's more about leading, following, additional moves, styling, or just more information about the basics, the options are plentiful. It might be best to do a search online for your particular area with the words "tango" and your home city. See what you come up with. Ballrooms, social dance clubs, community centers, and freelance instructors are all part of what you might find. It's time to get out there on the dance floor and tango with the best of them. See where this dance might take you. Have fun, stay emotional, and continue your learning. It'll provide a lifetime of entertainment!

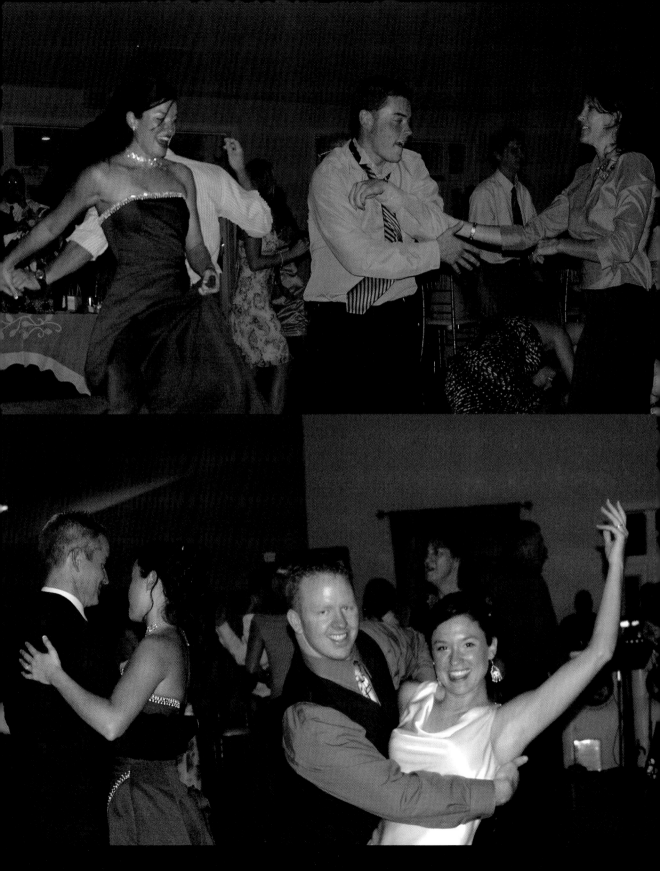

12

Picture Yourself *Dancing at Your Wedding*

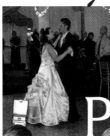

PICTURE YOUR wedding reception. You and your now husband are standing off of the floor, waiting to be introduced to your family and friends as husband and wife. As soon as you are introduced, your song is started by your deejay or band—the song that you will remember for the rest of your life as your wedding song. How do you select this song? How long do you dance once you are out on the floor? What dance is best for this occasion? Do you really need hundreds of dollars in dance lessons to look decent out there? Are there any quick tricks or tips you should know? All these questions and more will be answered in this section. Learning to dance for a wedding is one of those motivators that is often discussed and much less frequently acted upon. Once the expenses start cropping up, the leftover funds for dance lessons continue to dwindle. Don't let your budget or your busy schedule keep you from having a wonderfully memorable first dance at your wedding. Now that you have read and learned the basics of the nine dances taught in this book, you are armed and ready to make some informed decisions and step out with the right foot on the dance floor (as long as you are the follower!).

Dancing at Your Wedding

ANCING OF VARIOUS forms is a part of the vast majority of weddings. Some couples choose a theme for their music and dancing for their event, while others simply request the deejay or band play whatever is popular. With the dancing tools that you have learned in this text, a little bit of forethought, and some practice, you have the makings for a highly enjoyable and entertaining reception. Because the first dance is such a large part of your own experience as the bride or groom, it will be addressed by itself a bit later in this chapter.

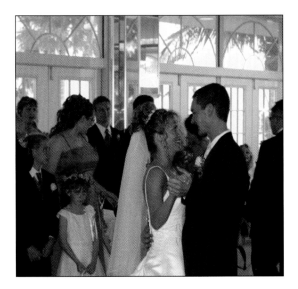

The Location

Although you can dance almost anywhere, please be sensitive to your surroundings and your guests. If possible, place the dance floor within the sight line of the vast majority of your guests. If by necessity you need to seat guests beyond the visual reach of the dance floor and festivities, try to arrange seating nearby so your guests can somewhat comfortably view such important events as the first dance, the father-daughter dance, and the mother-son dance. It's also recommended that you leave at least a foot between all edges of the dance floor and the nearest table. Dancers tend to spill off of the dance floor during the more lively tunes, whether they are freestyle dancing or couples dancing, and that extra little buffer of space usually gives them enough of a heads up before they hit someone.

The Music

Whether you have a band or a deejay, take the time before the event to acclimate them a little bit to your crowd. If you know the crowd consists of slow starters, let the deejay or emcee know—sometimes they have some tricks to get the crowd going. If there is a particular type of music that really gets your cousins out on the dance floor, you should also educate your entertainment crew. Everyone has a better time when the correct music is played. Just in case, speaking from our own experience, provide a written list of the important names in the wedding party and how they are pronounced, as well as songs that you definitely want played or not played at your wedding. Don't be afraid of line dances, such as the Electric Slide. They can be invaluable for getting your crowd going. Just remember, your guests are taking their cues from you—if you aren't participating, they probably won't either.

Dance Lessons for the Guests

We have participated in several wedding celebrations where the bride and groom incorporated a dance lesson for their guests into the festivities. Before you scream "budget" on this one, we have found that it can actually save you some money on your bar bill if you are providing an open bar for your guests. Bored guests tend to drink more heavily, and their biggest beverage time is while you are otherwise occupied with photographs and signing wedding licenses.

A great lesson while you and your wedding party are tied up with the pictures can set the tone for the rest of the celebration. We've seen brides and grooms take this opportunity to introduce a theme for the event that might have otherwise been foreign to the guests at large. For instance, we've taught a salsa lesson prior to a Latin-themed dinner reception for which the bride had hired a great salsa band. The guests knew enough basics to hit the floor and boogie with the bride and groom.

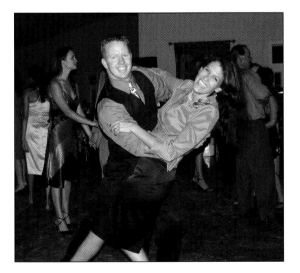

This group was especially clever because they allowed for enough time while the guests were being seated for the bridal party to have a mini-lesson in a side room after the main group lesson for the guests. That way, everyone was on the same foot, locals and out-of-town guests alike.

We've also seen the dance lesson incorporated into the reception following the first dances, but the success of this strategy depends on the bride and groom and immediate wedding party leading their guests onto the dance floor in participation.

Line dances or party dances can really get your party going if done correctly. These also depend on your participation and your immediate wedding party's participation. Yes, there is more to party dancing than the chicken dance and the Macarena. Ask your deejay, and if he seems to be out of ideas, look for a local line-dance instructor. Most line-dance instructors have material for more than just country music. The line dances give your crowd an opportunity to shake a leg in a structured format without the pressure of couples dancing. A good instructor or deejay really makes the difference here.

Make sure the instruction is in short spurts and not for long periods—this will also let you gauge your audience. Another key ingredient is the quality of the group instruction. A deadpan or overwhelmed instructor can be disastrous for your reception. When you are considering a group lesson at your wedding, attend a group class or two of the instructors you are interviewing. You are looking for someone with charisma, who is comfortable with a microphone, and who can put a large, diverse group at ease while still teaching them some dancing. Be choosy—it's your special event!

The First Dance

AHHHH, THE FIRST dance; your first opportunity to showcase each other as husband and wife following the ceremony has arrived. You have a variety of options that fall on a spectrum somewhere between walking onto the dance floor, embracing, and leaning into each other while swaying, and learning an elaborately choreographed routine that you spent months preparing for the three minutes of fame during your first dance. Typically, the bride and groom are first-time dancers and simply want to look like they know what they're doing out on the dance floor.

Without making you into an expert, these next couple of pages should provide you with enough insight into the dance and how to pull it off to make you look smooth without years of instruction. It's understood that you are event-driven, but don't overlook some basic factors that can help make your dance a success. Whether you're dancing a

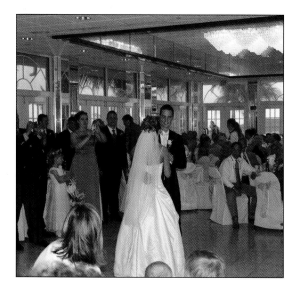

lead-and-follow dance, choreographing your dance, or having an instructor help you, there are certain elements that you should consider. Following is a listing of some of what you'll need to think about regarding your music and your dance:

▶ **The song. Pick two or three "first dance" songs and work with them during your dance lessons. You might find that one song is much better to dance to than another as you practice your steps. An extensive song database can be found at www.PictureYourselfDancing.com.**

▶ **The speed of the song. Is it too slow, too fast, or just right? Dancing with your partner to the speed of the song is important because you'll want to go with a speed you're comfortable with.**

▶ **The length of the song. Shorter is better! If you're able to, try to keep the song *less than* three minutes. If it's a band playing this might be difficult, but if it's a deejay, it's possible to have him fade it. The old saying about there being "too much of a good thing" is true when it comes to the first dance. A long song makes everyone uncomfortable, not just the bride and groom. Always leave your audience wanting more!**

▶ **The words of the song. Make sure you're both comfortable with the words that are used in your song. Don't just pick one because you like the beat. Try to find a song that you'll always remember and that either fits your relationship or fits what you'd like it to become. Does** the song just make you want to say "Awwwwwww!" every time you hear it? If so, you might have found the perfect song for the two of you.

▶ Size of the dance floor. How much space do you have to dance and where will your audience be? This is critical in choosing your dance and picking your moves. You don't want to do a very small dance (not much moving) on a very large floor. By the same token, when you are dancing your first dance please be aware of where your guests are. If they are on three sides or completely surround the dance floor, please dance accordingly. Your family and friends would like to see your glowing faces for at least part of the dance.

▶ What you're wearing. You should always practice in something similar to what you'll be wearing at your reception. If the bride is wearing a strapless dress, she should practice in one so you'll both know the limitations. Ladies, it's

imperative that you practice in the shoes you'll be wearing or ones that are strikingly similar in height, feel, and heel size. Guys, if you'll be wearing a coat the night of your dance, you should practice in one.

▶ The entrance. How will you walk onto the dance floor, and will it be before the song or after the song starts? For many songs, it might be best to walk out arm in arm after your music starts and do a walking underarm turn and come back to a quick, romantic kiss. Your entrance will appear choreographed and will capture your audience's attention while filling up some very valuable seconds.

When to Start

You should at least start thinking about the dancing at your wedding, the first dance and otherwise, in the earliest stages of your wedding plans. Whether you want to have dancing at all will probably play an important role in your reception location as well as the time of day of your wedding.

If any dancing beyond the cursory first dance and father-daughter dance is not on your wish list at all, a brunch reception would probably suit you well and save you quite a bit of money in catering. However, if you want an evening reception with a rocking deejay on a Saturday night in June, you will need to plan further in advance and budget accordingly for everything. Chances are you won't be getting as many discounts from your vendors.

That being said, you do not need to start taking lessons the instant you set a date. Yes, you definitely want to allow yourself enough time, and most instructors recommend at least three months.

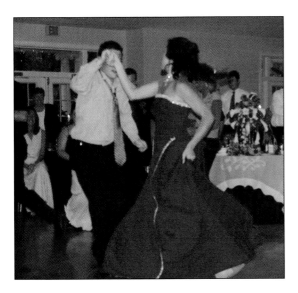

However, we have taught several couples to dance the day before their wedding, and countless more the week before their wedding. There's nothing like a deadline to make people move! Yes, those last-minute learners were happy with their results at their receptions, but we don't recommend the extreme last minute to anyone. It is very nerve-wracking. The only up side is when you leave it to the last minute, although you don't really have much time to develop good muscle memory, you certainly don't have time to develop any bad dance habits either.

If you plan to learn from a video or DVD, plan to start learning and adjusting to your music about six weeks in advance. This allows for plenty of practice time and tweaking of your music selection if necessary. If you are already under the wire time-wise, go for private lessons with a reputable instructor in your area. If the instructor is worth his salt, he should be able to polish the two of you up in a handful of sessions.

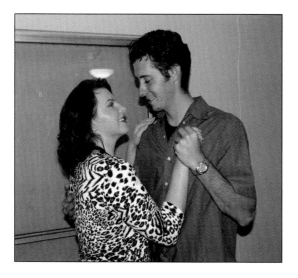

Who Needs to Know What

As you coordinate with your wedding professionals, keep the channels of communication open. If you are doing a choreographed first dance or are at least planning to do a true lead-and-follow dance with actual moves other than the lean-'n-sway, you need to alert your deejay, videographer, photographer, and wedding coordinator or the manager/head server at your reception (if you have one). You will also need to let these same people know if you are planning to have a dance lesson or have a dancing crowd attending. These are all things that will impact the manner in which the aforementioned wedding professionals will conduct their business throughout your event.

Your photographer and videographer will have much more to work with and should be able to provide you with a higher quality and more interesting end product, your deejay will probably do a little research based on your information and modify his playlist to better suit your party, and your wedding coordinator or your event planner for the reception facility might have a different recommendation for the layout or the food and beverage services you are providing for your guests. Trust us, if you have selected quality vendors, these people will be genuinely excited to be associated with a dancing wedding reception. Your guests will have more fun, whether or not they are dancing, and you will most likely have a better overall experience.

Do not forget to coordinate with your groom and your father as well as your dance instructor, brides! There is important information that these individuals need in order to create the ultimate first dance for you. Although it is perfectly acceptable and appropriate for you to maintain a sense of mystery about your dress, you will need to give your dance partners and your instructor some general ideas.

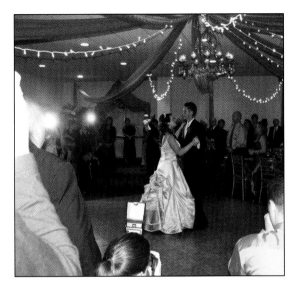

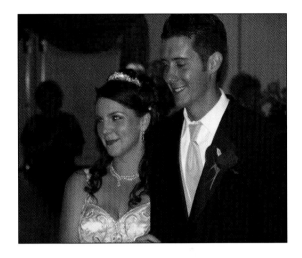

For instance, if your dress is a sheath or mermaid-style dress, you will be gorgeous, but you will not be taking very many long steps, so waltz might not be your best option for a first dance. If your gown is off the shoulder, you will also need to let your partners and instructor know because this will inhibit your ability to lift your arm, and your turns will need to be modified accordingly by the choreographer. For those of you with strapless gowns, let your partners know that they need to be careful. We have seen brides come flying out of their tops courtesy of an overly zealous dip. It was hilarious for everyone but the bride. If the groom practices being careful beforehand, he has a better chance of success when he is nervous or has had a few drinks.

Final Thoughts on Dancing and Weddings

As you plan and prepare for your big day, don't lose sight of the fact that your first dance, toasts, dress, flowers, music, and food are meant to be a celebration of your marriage to each other. Not one of the previously mentioned items should

overshadow your union as a couple. Our three final tips are given in an effort to maintain the integrity of your dance and make it just another wonderful part of your big day that will live for some time in your memory and the memories of your guests as a beautiful moment that they shared with you.

▶ **Practice as if it's the big day. Grooms should practice in a jacket and dress shoes. Brides should practice in a long skirt or their crinoline, if possible, and their wedding shoes. To protect your shoes from smudges or scuffs, cover them with athletic socks while they are on your feet. If you plan to wear a veil during your dance (not recommended), be sure to practice with this as well. Once you are fairly comfortable with your steps, try to practice in front of a friend to prepare you for dancing in front of an audience.**

As silly as it might sound, if you plan to drink at your reception, practice your dance after a few drinks. You want to at least be aware of what you'll look like, and you might need to modify some of the moves.

Finally, practice in front of a camera and/or video camera, especially if you're going to have a photographer or videographer at your wedding. At the end of your wedding, you're going to have three things: your memories, your photos, and your video. Your memories will be shaped by the two things that are tangible (the photos and the video), so you really ought to invest some time in front of them before your debut.

▶ Don't fight with each other. Take it easy on each other during lessons and practice. As they say, it takes two to tango, and when something goes wrong, it is rarely one person's fault. You are a team and need to work together. Never compare yourself to one another or to the instructor. This should be a fun part of your wedding plans, so no fights!

▶ Be honest. Be honest with yourselves, your band leader/deejay, your dance instructor, and anyone else who is involved in making your wedding decisions. If you don't want to dance the entire song, don't. If you don't like a certain move, don't do it. If you want to change songs, do it. It's your day and your dance; you should feel comfortable.

Now that you and your future spouse have all the tools, hit the dance floor and make some memories! This is a special occasion into which hours upon hours of preparation and planning have been poured. If you don't know how to dance, wow your friends and family and learn. If you shake a leg effectively at your wedding, you will remember it for years to come with pride.

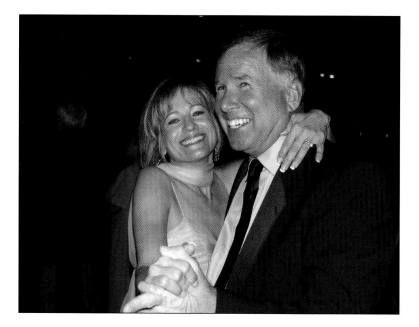

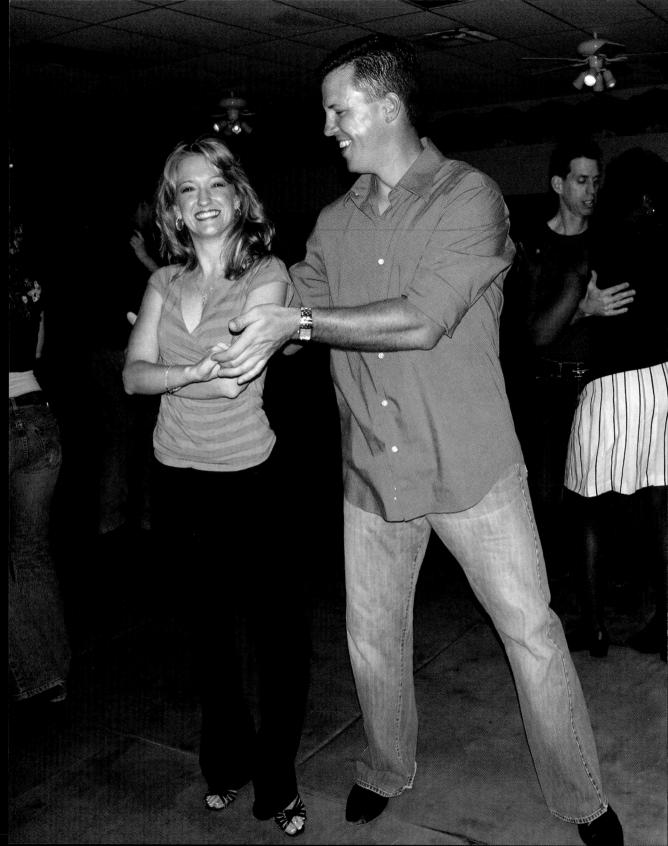

13

Picture Yourself

Dancing for Life

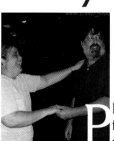

PICTURE YOURSELF out on your favorite dance floor. It might be your local pub, a dance studio, a posh country club, or a country-western nightclub. The floor is empty except for you and your dance partner. The bartender is wiping down the bar; the staff is starting to clean up around the perimeter of the dance floor. You and your partner are savoring the last strains of the dance as the venue closes down. The two of you have danced the night away after learning the basics of nine different dances. There wasn't a song that you couldn't dance to, be it a waltz, cha-cha, swing, or two-step. You mastered the basics, used great lead-and-follow techniques, and had a great time on the dance floor. You used key concepts emphasized throughout this text and the accompanying DVD to learn a brand-new activity from the ground up. In this chapter, take a moment to review the key concepts that you have learned throughout the book. Use the summary tools and references for further information as you define your own personal dance tastes and further your dance education.

Key Points, Phrases, and Lists to Remember

FOLLOWING IS A COMPILATION of some of the most useful information mentioned in this book. Be sure to keep these things in mind as you embark upon your many dance outings from here on out. First, there are two main rules that everyone needs to remember:

1. Ladies are always right! (Ladies *always* start with their right foot.)

2. Guys always get what's left! (Guys *always* start with their left foot.)

Partner Etiquette

Partner etiquette is critical because it takes two of you to make this work. Some important thoughts include:

1. Don't give unsolicited advice to your partner.

2. Trust your partner.

3. Thank your partner after each dance.

Floor Etiquette

Floor etiquette is equally as important and has four main elements to it:

1. Always introduce yourself when dancing with someone new.

2. Be aware of your surroundings.

3. Apologize or excuse yourself if a collision occurs on the dance floor.

4. Know the correct placement for each dance.

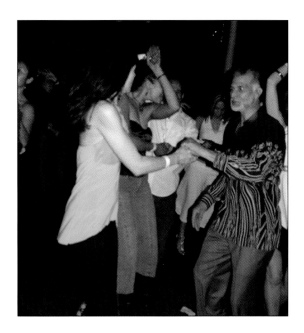

Four Connection Points

There are four connection points that are critical to creating the perfect dance frame. The dance frame is much like a picture frame in that it is meant to hold the subject in a position that allows for optimal viewing. The four connection points in their most elementary form include:

1. Leader's left hand and follower's right hand

2. Leader's right palm on the follower's left shoulder-blade

3. Follower's left elbow on the leader's right elbow

4. Follower's left hand on the inside edge of the leader's right shoulder

Five Basic Foot Positions

The five basic foot positions describe almost every step that you'll take in dancing. If you learned them early on, you found the foot placements to be extremely easy as each dance was taught. The five positions include:

1. First (feet together)

2. Second (feet shoulder-width apart)

3. Third and Extended Third (heel to instep)

4. Fourth (passing of feet)

5. Fifth and Extended Fifth (heel to toe)

Six Basic Dance Positions

The six basic dance positions were used throughout this book and describe the type of positions you're most likely to encounter when social dancing. The six positions and the basics of the dances you'll find them in most as you continue your dancing include:

1. Open (cha-cha, salsa)

2. One-hand hold (cha-cha, swing, salsa, West coast swing, hustle)

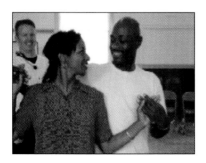

3. Two-hand hold (cha-cha, waltz, swing, salsa, West coast swing, hustle)

4. Closed (all dances in this book)

5. Promenade (waltz, two-step, swing, tango, hustle)

6. Sweetheart (waltz, two-step, hustle)

Seven Essential Steps

Seven essential steps have guided your learning and are critical to the success of each and every dance. Without a thorough understanding of the steps listed below, you would have difficulty learning the basics of the dances. The dances where the basics and variations of the basics can be found are listed next to each essential step.

1. Walking-steps (waltz, two-step, tango, West coast swing)

2. Side-steps (cha-cha, waltz, swing, slow dance, salsa)

3. Step-touches (slow dance, West coast swing)

4. Tap-steps (slow dance, tango, West coast swing)

5. Triple-steps (cha-cha, swing, salsa, West coast swing, hustle)

6. Rock-steps (cha-cha, swing, salsa, slow dance, tango, hustle)

7. Anchor-steps (West coast swing)

Eight Directional Possibilities

Eight directional possibilities quickly and easily point you in the right direction when determining where to step. The eight directions include (from the top of the spectrum to the right and all the way around):

▶ Forward

▶ Front-right

▶ Right

▶ Back-right

▶ Backward

▶ Back-left

▶ Left

▶ Front-left

Keep all of these things in mind because they're all critical success factors in your early stages of dance. Building the right foundation will dramatically increase your beginner to intermediate to advanced dancer timeframe.

Three Main Rules for Leaders and Followers

The following table shows the three main rules for leaders and followers in social dancing.

Followers	Leaders
Don't hang on!	Don't let her hang on!
Don't let go!	Don't let her go!
Don't think!	Don't make her think!

Dancing and Practicing for Fun

NOW THAT YOU'VE completed the book, you're probably looking for fun ways to practice the dances. That being said, we've put together a small collection of the best drills found in the book to practice each of your dances. Although some of them were found in specific dances, each of the ones in the following sections can be done with any dance, so make the most of your learning and enjoy practicing your new dance skills.

Chair Dancing

This is one that you can do right there while you're sitting in a chair somewhere. You'll focus on the steps and the timing of each dance—try each one this way. As you sit, you'll first put your feet in the ready position, then you'll start taking very small, discrete steps in place while you say the basic to yourself. For example, doing two-step, you'd be saying "quick-quick, slow, slow...quick-quick, slow, slow," while your feet are doing the steps in place. It's a good idea to practice a few minutes here and a few minutes there, but not for long sessions because you'll wear yourself out while you're sitting.

Shadow Dancing

This is another one you can try on your own, just to reinforce the basics of each dance. Dance through everything you just learned, or at a minimum, the basics of each dance without a partner—just imagine your partner is there doing the steps with you as you dance along. See how long you can last without messing up, stopping, or getting off beat.

Try to run through the leads and/or follows and footwork for all of the dances and moves in your repertoire, and it will dramatically improve your long-term memory as well as your muscle memory.

Speed Dancing

This is one where you and your partner will test out several different speeds of each dance—slow, medium, fast, super fast, and so on. With or without music, this drill is fun because it allows you to test your limits in both directions while building control and muscle memory.

Blindfolded Dancing

This is a fun way to practice both the leading and the following elements. Leaders, you'll get to do this one too! Practice each dance three different ways:

1. With the leaders blindfolded

2. With the followers blindfolded

3. With both partners blindfolded

This exercise will certainly reinforce the importance of nonverbal communication through effective leading and following. Note: Leaders, don't blindfold yourself on progressive dances!

Partnership Pointers

MUCH OF WHAT IS LISTED in this section is taught throughout the book, but not in a condensed and consolidated form. In dance, and also in life, these are 10 things that everyone should know:

1. Focus on the "what" rather than the "who" when looking into something being right or wrong. Try to work through troubleshooting options while you practice. (Besides, now that you've been through the rest of the book, you know who's always right!)

2. Dancing is very logical and "event driven." Everything happens for a reason! As the old saying goes, "For every action, there is an equal and opposite reaction."

3. The game "Follow the Leader" works when the follower is led gently and with confidence. Leaders, don't second guess yourselves, but don't force the lead either.

4. Be considerate of your partner or those you're working with. If you recognize a problem, find a way to work together to fix the problem, not the person or the people. Make sure you separate the two!

5. Every dance partnership is a two-way street that's split right down the middle when it comes to responsibility. Both leaders and followers have their own rules and responsibilities in every dance (as we covered in each of the chapters). If one partner fails, both do.

6. Sensitivity is key! Think before you speak, and certainly before you blame. There's a good chance that you might be able to make a change that makes the difference. Try to adjust something that you're doing before you attempt to change your partner.

7. Good partnerships require work. Work to understand everything that's going on so you can help focus on any problems that come up.

8. Take the time to celebrate small successes as you learn to dance. Small successes are critical milestones along the path of much larger ones.

9. Feelings are important! (Don't overlook this point.) It's been said that we often judge others not by who they are, but by who we are when we are with them. Make your partner feel great, and you, in turn, will be judged accordingly. People remember feelings much more clearly than they remember specific words or statements.

10. Every interaction on the dance floor is a mini-relationship. The respect, courtesy, patience, understanding, and connection that one gives to their partner are all symbolic of what someone could be like off the floor. You project the type of person you are by how you handle yourself during the dance.

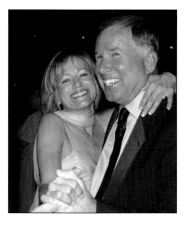

The Nine-Dance Matrix

Dance	Social Dance Subculture	Time Signature	Tempo	Basic Count	How to Say It
Slow dance	Latin, ballroom, country, swing	4/4	Slow	1, 2, 3, 4	Step, touch, step, touch
Waltz	Ballroom, country	3/4	Slow	1, 2, 3, 4, 5, 6	One, two, three, four, five, six
Two-step	Country	4/4	Medium/fast	1, 2, 3, 5	Quick, quick, slow, slow
Swing	Ballroom, country, swing	4/4	Fast	1, 3, 5, 6	Step, step, rock-step
Cha-cha	Ballroom, country, Latin	4/4	Medium	1, 2, 3 & 4, 5, 6, 7 & 8	One, two, cha-cha-cha
Salsa	Ballroom, Latin	4/4	Fast	1, 2, 3, 5, 6, 7	Quick, quick, slow, quick, quick, slow
Hustle	Ballroom, country, swing	4/4	Medium	And-1, 2, 3	Quick, quick, slow, slow or and-one, two, three
West coast swing	Country, ballroom, swing	4/4	Medium	1, 2, 3, 4, 5 & 6	Walk, walk, tap- (or triple-) step, anchor-step
Tango	Ballroom, Latin	4/4	Medium	1, 3, 5, 6, 7	T - A - N-G-O or one, two, tan-go-close

Dance Cheat Sheets

THE MATRIX on the previous page is a quick way to compare the various dances. The next pages provide a succinct synopsis of each of the dances that you have learned. You can use these abbreviated descriptions as a type of cheat sheet as you navigate between the dances or look for a quick refresher before hitting the dance floor.

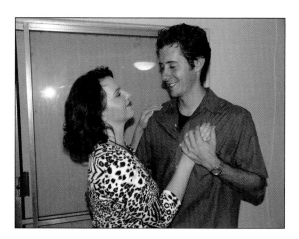

Slow Dance

► **Type. Slow dance is slow and romantic. You will see it at any and every occasion with dancing. It is found in the ballroom, country, Latin, and swing dance subcultures.**

► **Timing. The music is either 2/4 or 4/4 timing.**

► **Tempo. Slow.**

► **Basic rhythm. Step, touch, step, touch, with one step for each beat of music.**

► **Count. 1, 2, 3, 4.**

► **Characteristics. A spot dance with simple footwork and a very smooth and controlled look.**

► **Seen at. Weddings, nightclubs, reunions, cruises.**

► **Practice songs. For updated song lists for each style of dance and more tips and pointers for each dance, go to www.PictureYourselfDancing.com or www.ShawnTrautman.com.**

Waltz

► **Type. The waltz is a smooth and graceful ballroom and country-western dance typified by rise and fall movement.**

► **Timing. The music is 3/4 timing.**

► **Tempo. Slow (with the exception of Viennese waltz, which is extremely fast).**

► **Basic rhythm. Step, step, close, step, step, close, with one step for each beat of music.**

► **Count. 1, 2, 3, 4, 5, 6.**

► **Characteristics. Progressive with a very smooth and controlled look. When executed correctly, the couple appears to float around the floor.**

► **Seen at. Ballrooms, occasionally country-western nightclubs, and weddings.**

▶Practice songs. For updated song lists for each style of dance and more tips and pointers for each dance, go to www.PictureYourselfDancing.com or www.ShawnTrautman.com.

Two-Step

▶Type. Two-step is a country-western dance with a smooth, driving beat.

▶Timing. The music is 4/4 timing.

▶Tempo. Medium to fast.

▶Basic rhythm. Quick, quick, slow, slow, with each quick being one beat of music and each slow being two beats of music.

▶Count.1, 2, 3, (hold 4), 5, (hold 6).

▶Characteristics. Progressive dance with a long stride and a level top line. The feet glide just above the floor. The two-step has a light and fun attitude.

▶Seen at. Country-western events and nightclubs.

▶Practice songs. For updated song lists for each style of dance and more tips and pointers for each dance, go to www.PictureYourselfDancing.com or www.ShawnTrautman.com.

Swing

▶Type. Swing is a fun dance that has its own dance subculture but has also been adopted by the ballroom and country-western subcultures.

▶Timing. The music is 4/4 timing.

▶Tempo. Fast.

▶Basic rhythm. Slow, slow, quick, quick or step, step, rock-step, with each quick being one beat of music and each slow being two beats of music.

▶Count. 1, (hold 2), 3, (hold 4), 5, 6.

▶Characteristics. The swing is a spot dance with lilt and circular movement. Rather than dancing around the circumference of the dance floor, the couples rotate back and forth in place. Swing is a fun, lively, jazzy, and upbeat dance.

▶Seen at. Weddings, nightclubs, reunions, cruises, country-western events, and ballrooms.

▶Practice songs. For updated song lists for each style of dance and more tips and pointers for each dance, go to www.PictureYourselfDancing.com or http://www.ShawnTrautman.com.

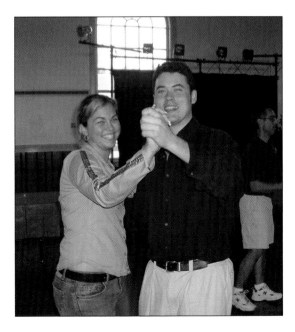

Cha-Cha

- ►Type. Cha-cha is a flirtatious and sassy Latin dance that has been adopted by the ballroom and country-western sub-cultures.

- ►Timing. The music is 4/4 timing.

- ►Tempo. Medium.

- ►Basic rhythm. Slow, slow, quick, quick, slow or step, step, cha-cha-cha, with each slow being one beat of music and each quick being half a beat of music.

- ►Count. 1, 2, 3, and 4.

- ►Characteristics. Cha-cha is a slotted dance with flirtatious Cuban motion. Small steps should be taken on the ball of the foot, followed by the heel being lowered in a controlled fashion to the floor. Alternating use of slow and staccato movements typify the dance.

- ►Seen at. Latin nightclubs, country-western events, and ballrooms.

- ►Practice songs. For updated song lists for each style of dance and more tips and pointers for each dance, go to www.PictureYourselfDancing.com or www.ShawnTrautman.com.

Salsa

- ►Type. Salsa is a hot and spicy Latin dance.

- ►Timing. The music is 4/4 timing.

- ►Tempo. Fast and faster. Eat your chili peppers before you dance this one!

- ►Basic rhythm. Quick, quick, slow, quick, quick, slow, with one quick for each beat of music and two beats of music for each slow.

- ►Count. 1, 2, 3, (hold 4), 5, 6, 7, (hold 8).

- ►Characteristics. Salsa is a spot dance with a smooth upper torso and a cooking lower body. Cuban motion is a large part of the salsa look. Small steps taken on the ball of the foot are key to mastery of salsa.

- ►Seen at. Weddings, Latin nightclubs, and ballrooms.

- ►Practice songs. For updated song lists for each style of dance and more tips and pointers for each dance, go to www.PictureYourselfDancing.com or www.ShawnTrautman.com.

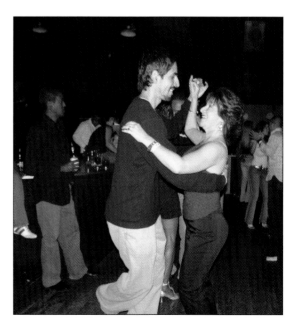

Hustle

- ▶ Type. Hustle is an American dance that is a derivative of swing. It has been adopted by the ballroom and country-western circuits. Although hustle is a type of swing dance, you will rarely see it at a swing event.

- ▶ Timing. The music is 4/4 timing.

- ▶ Tempo. Medium.

- ▶ Basic rhythm. Quick, quick, slow, slow, with each quick being half a beat of music and each slow being one beat of music. It is also counted "and-1, 2, 3."

- ▶ Count. And-1, 2, 3.

- ▶ Characteristics. Hustle is a smooth spot dance that is typified by an elastic lead-and-follow relationship in which the follower is almost constantly turning. The follower's footwork is marked by a rock-step on the quicks in each basic.

- ▶ Seen at. Weddings, nightclubs, and ballrooms.

- ▶ Practice songs. For updated song lists for each style of dance and more tips and pointers for each dance, go to www.PictureYourselfDancing.com or www.ShawnTrautman.com.

West Coast Swing

- ▶ Type. West coast swing is an advanced swing dance that has been adapted to match the blues and other popular rhythms and has been adopted by both ballroom and country subcultures.

- ▶ Timing. The music is 4/4 timing.

- ▶ Tempo. Medium.

- ▶ Basic rhythm. Walk, walk, tap-step (or triple-step), anchor-step. Each walk is one beat of music, each tap-step or triple-step is two beats (three steps to two beats of music), and the three steps of the anchor-step are two beats.

- ▶ Count. 1, 2, 3, 4 or (3 and 4), 5 and 6.

- ▶ Characteristics. West coast swing is the king of swing dances. It is the most difficult dance taught in this text. The moves are based on 6-, 8-, 10-, or 12-beat patterns. The dance is a completely lead-and-follow dance in which the woman is doing most of the movement but the man is the master of leverage.

- ▶ Seen at. West coast swing dances, swing dances, ballrooms, nightclubs, and country-western events.

- ▶ Practice songs. For updated song lists for each style of dance and more tips and pointers for each dance, go to www.PictureYourselfDancing.com or www.ShawnTrautman.com.

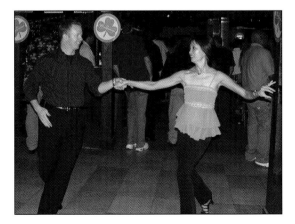

Tango

- ▶ **Type.** Tango is a Latin dance that has been championed by the ballroom sub-culture.

- ▶ **Timing.** The music is primarily 4/4 timing, but the earliest music was 2/4 timing.

- ▶ **Tempo.** Medium.

- ▶ **Basic rhythm.** Slow, slow, quick, quick, slow or step, step, tan-go-close, with each slow being two beats of music and each quick being one beat of music.

- ▶ **Count.** 1, (hold 2), 3, (hold 4), 5, 6, 7, (hold 8).

- ▶ **Characteristics.** Tango is a progressive dance marked by drama, catlike walks, a close hold, and bold, firm steps with lots of attitude. The tango is filled with passion expressed through sensual movements.

- ▶ **Seen at.** Ballrooms and some Latin nightclubs.

- ▶ **Practice songs.** For updated song lists for each style of dance and more tips and pointers for each dance, go to www.PictureYourselfDancing.com or www.ShawnTrautman.com.

Next Steps (Continued Learning)

T O CONTINUE YOUR learning after you're comfortable with the practicing, you might choose to do more reading, take a look at more videos (DVDs), or learn from a dance pro near you. Regardless, the following information will help assist you with your next steps because it focuses on helping social dancers like yourself.

Dance Resources Online

For a complete listing of dance-related resources, including videos/DVDs, updated song lists for each style of dance, a wedding song database, national and international dance organizations, professional memberships, and more tips and pointers for each dance, go to either of the following:

▶ www.PictureYourselfDancing.com

▶ www.ShawnTrautman.com

Private Lessons/ Choosing an Instructor

You might find that you're now in need of some personal attention and you'd like to find a dance instructor to help you. Before choosing a dance instructor, you must first consider how proficient you want to become and what type of dancing you want to do. If you just want to get out and have fun with the dances, then you might not need to go to the top ballroom in the area when an instructor at the local community center or the local country nightclub could easily and much more affordably show you the ropes. Conversely, if you want to get into couples dancing as a serious hobby or for competitive reasons, you would want

to look for professional qualifications and backgrounds and someone with a dance style that you'd like to emulate.

As you look for the right instructor, don't just look for how someone dances. Excellent dancers are usually perceived and considered to be great instructors, whether they've ever taught anyone or not. Get recommendations. Sometimes they are also great instructors and sometimes they're not. One has very little to do with the other. The ability to communicate effectively on an interpersonal level is a quality that should be sought when selecting an instructor. It's best to find an instructor who is encouraging, who makes you feel comfortable, who conveys the information you need in a timely fashion, and who doesn't come across as someone who's on a completely different level than yourself. Yes, the instructor needs to know what they're talking about, but they do not need to hold a certain number of dance competition titles or be members of every known dance association to be qualified. There are plenty of wonderful instructors out there who don't dance competitively, and there are many excellent dance competitors whose passion is in dancing and not teaching.

A last consideration for the instructor relates to the cost and what you have budgeted for your undertaking. Some ballrooms, studios, and instructors allow you to pay by the hour, while others have lesson packages available that guide you through well-versed curriculums. Whichever road you take, make it an enjoyable trip and you'll want to continue with it.

Final Thoughts from Shawn and Joanna

CONGRATULATIONS! You made it! You survived 13 fun-filled chapters of dance instruction, tips, tricks, and drills. Hopefully by this point in the book you've mastered, or at least been exposed to and attempted, the various concepts that are critical to your success as a social dancer, from floor etiquette, to musical intelligence, to some great basic dance moves. We hope you've enjoyed the journey.

We put a lot from our combined experiences into this text. We are serious about the followers using proper dance frame to defend themselves against bad breath and overly-friendly dance partners, just as we are speaking from experience when we emphasize the importance of introducing oneself prior to dancing with someone. We can't count the number of times we've been out dancing socially and complete strangers have come up to one of us, demanded a dance, and never even bothered to introduce themselves. Social dance is self-defining —it is a rhythmic, movement-based activity that is defined by interpersonal communication. Enjoy it— we do! There are myriad possibilities as far as activities, venues, lessons, and even competitions that are now open to you.

As you continue dancing, we hope you take the firm foundation that you obtained through the *Picture Yourself Dancing* book and DVD and grow from it. There are many opportunities out there,

from DVDs to group lessons to specialized private instruction. When the moment presents itself, seize the chance and step out on the dance floor. We hope a lifetime of dancing is in your future!

All our best to you. Maybe we'll see you out on the dance floor soon!

—Shawn and Joanna Trautman

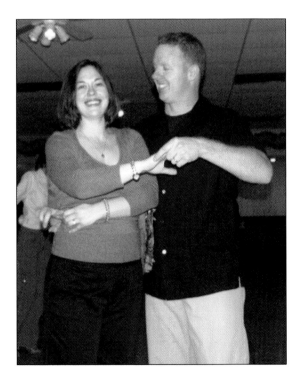

Index

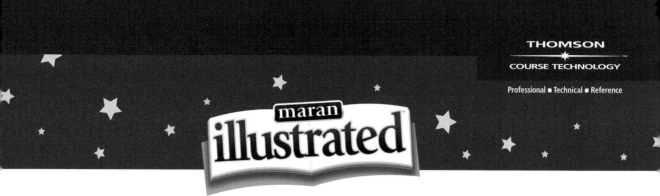

If you enjoy the visual style of learning, then check out these one-of-a-kind guides from the award-winning maranGraphics group!

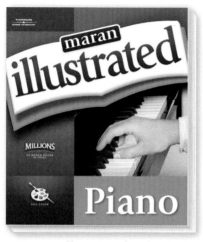

Maran Illustrated™ Piano
ISBN: 1-59200-864-X ■ $24.99 U.S.

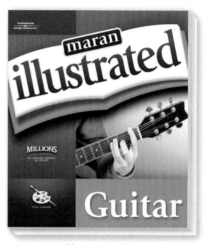

Maran Illustrated™ Guitar
ISBN: 1-59200-860-7 ■ $24.99 U.S.

Whether you want to play a few songs for your family in the living room or you aspire to become a serious musician, *Maran Illustrated Piano* is the ideal guide to help you reach your goal. You will learn the best way to perform each task as you learn your new skill while the full-color photographs, music examples and clear, step-by-step instructions walk you through each step from beginning to end. Thorough topic introductions and useful tips provide additional information and advice to help enhance your piano learning experience. *Maran Illustrated Piano* is packed with essential information for those who are sitting down in front of a piano for the first time, and provide more experienced players with a refresher course on the basics and the opportunity to add more advanced techniques to their repertoire. *Maran Illustrated Piano* costs less than the price of one private piano lesson and will be a permanent resource that provides years of enjoyment.

Whether you want to play a few songs with your family around the campfire or you aspire to become a serious musician or rock star, *Maran Illustrated Guitar* offers a unique, visual guide for learning to play the guitar. The full-color photographs, music examples and clear, step-by-step instructions walk you through each step from beginning to end. Thorough topic introductions and useful tips provide additional information and advice to help enhance your guitar experience. *Maran Illustrated Guitar* is packed with essential information for readers who are picking up a guitar for the first time, and also provides more experienced players with a refresher course on the basics and the opportunity to add more advanced techniques to their repertoire. *Maran Illustrated Guitar* costs less than the price of one private guitar lesson, and will be a permanent resource that provides years of enjoyment.

Check out the entire list of Maran Illustrated guides at www.courseptr.com

Call 1-888-270-9300 to order ■ Order online at www.courseptr.com

License Agreement/Notice of Limited Warranty

By opening the sealed disc container in this book, you agree to the following terms and conditions. If, upon reading the following license agreement and notice of limited warranty, you cannot agree to the terms and conditions set forth, return the unused book with unopened disc to the place where you purchased it for a refund.

License:

The enclosed software is copyrighted by the copyright holder(s) indicated on the software disc. You are licensed to copy the software onto a single computer for use by a single user and to a backup disc. You may not reproduce, make copies, or distribute copies or rent or lease the software in whole or in part, except with written permission of the copyright holder(s). You may transfer the enclosed disc only together with this license, and only if you destroy all other copies of the software and the transferee agrees to the terms of the license. You may not decompile, reverse assemble, or reverse engineer the software.

Notice of Limited Warranty:

The enclosed disc is warranted by Thomson Course Technology PTR to be free of physical defects in materials and workmanship for a period of sixty (60) days from end user's purchase of the book/disc combination. During the sixty-day term of the limited warranty, Thomson Course Technology PTR will provide a replacement disc upon the return of a defective disc.

Limited Liability:

THE SOLE REMEDY FOR BREACH OF THIS LIMITED WARRANTY SHALL CONSIST ENTIRELY OF REPLACEMENT OF THE DEFECTIVE DISC. IN NO EVENT SHALL THOMSON COURSE TECHNOLOGY PTR OR THE AUTHOR BE LIABLE FOR ANY OTHER DAMAGES, INCLUDING LOSS OR CORRUPTION OF DATA, CHANGES IN THE FUNCTIONAL CHARACTERISTICS OF THE HARDWARE OR OPERATING SYSTEM, DELETERIOUS INTERACTION WITH OTHER SOFTWARE, OR ANY OTHER SPECIAL, INCIDENTAL, OR CONSEQUENTIAL DAMAGES THAT MAY ARISE, EVEN IF THOMSON COURSE TECHNOLOGY PTR AND/OR THE AUTHOR HAS PREVIOUSLY BEEN NOTIFIED THAT THE POSSIBILITY OF SUCH DAMAGES EXISTS.

Disclaimer of Warranties:

THOMSON COURSE TECHNOLOGY PTR AND THE AUTHOR SPECIFICALLY DISCLAIM ANY AND ALL OTHER WARRANTIES, EITHER EXPRESS OR IMPLIED, INCLUDING WARRANTIES OF MERCHANTABILITY, SUITABILITY TO A PARTICULAR TASK OR PURPOSE, OR FREEDOM FROM ERRORS. SOME STATES DO NOT ALLOW FOR EXCLUSION OF IMPLIED WARRANTIES OR LIMITATION OF INCIDENTAL OR CONSEQUENTIAL DAMAGES, SO THESE LIMITATIONS MIGHT NOT APPLY TO YOU.

Other:

This Agreement is governed by the laws of the State of Massachusetts without regard to choice of law principles. The United Convention of Contracts for the International Sale of Goods is specifically disclaimed. This Agreement constitutes the entire agreement between you and Thomson Course Technology PTR regarding use of the software.